FAST Your WAY TO HEALTH

FAST Your WAY TO HEALTH

Lee Bueno

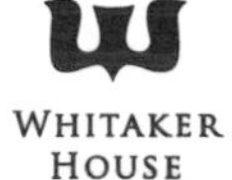

WHITAKER HOUSE

Note: This book is not intended to provide medical advice or to take the place of medical advice and treatment from your personal physician. Neither the publisher nor the author takes any responsibility for any possible consequences from any action taken by any person reading or following the information in this book. Always consult your physician or other qualified health care professional before undertaking any change in your physical regimen, whether fasting, diet, medications, or exercise.

FAST YOUR WAY TO HEALTH

To contact the author, write:
Lee Bueno
Buenos Amigos
P.O. Box 1675
Temecula, CA 92593

ISBN-13: 978-0-88368-657-7 • ISBN-10: 0-88368-657-0
Printed in the United States of America

Whitaker House
1030 Hunt Valley Circle
New Kensington, PA 15068
www.whitakerhouse.com

Library of Congress Cataloging-in-Publication Data

Bueno-Aguer, Lee, 1936–
Fast your way to health / by Lee Bueno-Aguer.
p. cm.
Includes bibliographical references (p.).
1. Fasting. 2. Fasting—Therapeutic use. I. Title.
BV5055 .B84 2001
248.4'7—dc21
2001000807

5 6 7 8 9 10 11 12 13 14 ꟺ 16 15 14 13 12 11 10 09

Contents

Foreword

As a doctor who specializes in the supervision of therapeutic fasting, I have witnessed the incredible self-healing potential of the body when the requirements of health are provided. Fasting is perhaps the most powerful tool in the health care arsenal and, when it is used appropriately, fasting is a safe and effective means of helping the body to heal itself. I suggest that individuals seek appropriate guidance before undertaking a fast.

—Alan Goldhamer, D.C.

Preface

Health is the most important factor in life. The wealthiest person invests his wealth first in his health—not in a bank that offers the highest dividends. All of a man's education, training, and experiences depend on the measure of health he enjoys.

This book has grown out of Lee's quest for knowledge and her subsequent rich experiences with fasting. She writes from a heart that yearns to help millions of sufferers in our sick society. Lee has the answers that many are earnestly seeking. This book is astounding, inspiring, and a great contribution to the welfare of all who seek to live in the best of health and enjoy life to its fullest.

—Costa S. Deir, M.D.H., Ph.D. Sc.D.

Acknowledgments

Long before this book became a reality, two editors contributed their writing skills and research to my original manuscript: Victoria Bidwell, an author who has her own publishing company, and Cecil Murphy, who has authored many books. Thanks also go to all those who helped, encouraged, and provided information and guidance; they are too numerous to mention individually.

A special thanks to our son, Chris, who contributed some helpful ideas, and our daughter, Kim, who gave me a perfect example of physical and emotional vitality with a ten-day fast. To my father, now past eighty years of age, who is rejoicing to see his daughter's book finally in print.

To my late husband, Elmer, about whom you will read throughout my book. Our lengthy, numerous discussions produced the encouragement that I needed to finish this project, which I enthusiastically started over eight years ago. His unselfish love and support, along with some ideas he allowed me to "steal," gave me the inspiration I needed. He's one in a million!

Introduction

You have in your hands a volume filled with exciting secrets—secrets of youthfulness, good health, healing, and spiritual victories. How our nation and our churches need to know these truths!

How did I become intrigued by fasting? As a dedicated minister's wife, I became perplexed by other people's seemingly unsolvable problems. The Bible recorded God's intervention in the cases of Moses, Esther, Nehemiah, Ezra, Daniel, Jehoshaphat, and many others as they prayed and fasted. Great men of God who changed nations—Luther, Wesley, Calvin, Finney, Knox, and others—were men who fasted and prayed.

But why fasting? Was it a sort of hunger strike to get God's attention? Was it to twist God's arm? No. Fasting intensifies prayer. A man who prays with fasting gives heaven notice that he is very serious about his petition. Prayer and fasting become the catalyst to change the impossible into victory.

Realizing I could not expect to have power over satanic forces if I did not have power over my appetite, I embarked on my first fast in the mid-1960s. By midafternoon I lay prostrate with a blinding headache and vomiting. I heartily agreed with my family that fasting was not for everyone—certainly not for me. A minister friend comforted me, "Some people pray more effectively on a full stomach."

But Jesus said in His Sermon on the Mount, *"When you fast"* (Matthew 6:16, 17), not "If you fast." After a few feeble attempts and failures, one day I announced, "I am going to fast! Please do not stop me!" I thought to myself, like Esther, *"If I perish, I perish!"* (Esther 4:16).

For a couple of days I practiced what I called "self-denial": consuming broth, crackers, weak tea—and then water only. I had not been a particularly healthy person. During my fast I experienced nausea, headaches, weakness, cramps, and hunger. But by the third or fourth day, I felt marvelous. I cooked for my family, joined friends as they ate out—and thoroughly enjoyed pure water. My body was cleansing itself; toxins had broken loose; and my stomach was on vacation.

Isaiah 58 became part of my daily Bible reading while I fasted. Verses six through twelve contain more promises of blessings than anywhere else in the Bible. Not only were there spiritual victories, but I had not realized how healthy I would become—and youthful and slim, too.

Fasting became a regular part of my life. At the beginning of each season of the year, I fasted ten, fourteen, or twenty-one days, one weekend each month, and two days each week. Spiritually, I witnessed miracles beyond my wildest dreams: people set free from drugs and alcohol, an insane woman delivered from a mental institution, a man healed of cancer, marriages restored, rebellious children reconciled to parents, incurable disease cured, and in 1973 a woman raised from the dead.

I'm so grateful that Lee Bueno is making us aware of a wonderful truth that has been hidden in the Bible for more than two thousand years. If you have never fasted before, Lee's book will launch you into an exciting physical and spiritual adventure.

—Pauline Harthern
Pastor's wife, Bible teacher,
and former columnist for
Charisma magazine

One

Something Is Terribly Wrong!

On this Monday morning, I was most definitely not in my favorite place or position! With my body as tense as a tightrope, I tried to fit into the curvature of a well-seasoned, black leather dentist's chair. My hands gripped the armrests until my knuckles turned white. I was in agony. Dr. Garcia had injected four doses of novocaine and didn't dare give more. As she drilled, the pain still darted down the left side of my jaw, deep into my neck. The drilling, gouging, and filling continued for two hours. Finally, Dr. Garcia finished. After making an appointment to return to her Tijuana office, I headed for our home in southern California.

On my drive home, the numbness from the novocaine in my jaw, lips, and the left side of my nose gradually began to subside. For years I had not been able to chew normally on that side of my mouth. The dentist had tried her best to save the badly decayed tooth. Soon I would know if she had succeeded.

Having dental work done "south of the border" was not new to us Buenos. For years we had lived as missionaries in Latin America. The dentists' prices, compared with those in the United States, made the two-hour drive to Tijuana worth the inconvenience. And this call had cost only twelve dollars—a real bargain!

As the familiar pain began to return, I wondered if Dr. Garcia had successfully repaired the tooth. A half bottle of aspirin and a couple of days later, I was gratefully free of pain, but my tooth still could not support any pressure. Although I was unable to use this salvaged tooth, at least it was capped and protected from further decay. Relieved that I had taken good care of myself, I turned my attention to our work in the ministry.

Trying to Ignore the Pain

That Friday morning, I awoke with excruciating pain at the base of my skull. I couldn't even lift my head from the pillow. "Oh, Elmer," I groaned. "It feels as if I have a head full of infection."

I thought back four days earlier to the visit with Dr. Garcia. The horror stories about the unsterilized instruments and primitive methods of Tijuana's doctors and dentists flashed through my head.

"No, it couldn't be!" I thought, trying to reassure myself. Not Dr. Garcia! She's so conscientious and meticulous. If my visit to Dr. Garcia's office had triggered this headache, it certainly wouldn't be her fault. I banished all negative thoughts from my mind and gulped down a couple of extra-strength aspirin. By 11:00 A.M., I was at my desk, hard at work. My positive thinking, painkillers, and mounds of correspondence in which to immerse myself had extinguished the burning pain in my head.

Several weeks later, however, strange twinges of pain and the gurgling, sloshing, swishing sounds in my head were too pronounced to ignore anymore. I had described this noisy sea in my head to my husband, and we had even joked about it. Immersed in denial, I refused to think that anything could be seriously wrong. I had no idea that these symptoms were signaling a threat upon my very life.

Despite my deep denial, my condition only worsened. While lying in bed at night, the pains became sharper and the noises louder. This time positive thinking, painkillers, and sprees of workaholism could not suppress the symptoms raging in my head. Whatever it was, it was getting worse. I finally faced the facts while my husband, Elmer, and I prepared to minister at a family camp in Prescott, Arizona. Reluctantly, I admitted I was too sick to go. Chris and Kim, our children, provided the music in my place. I remained at home—alone with the fearful twinges of pain and the sinister sea of sounds in my head.

Gripped by Fear

By the third night alone with only my symptoms for company, these unnerving pains and sounds progressed to a frightening stage. I could no longer deny the insidious whispering from my mind that something was terribly wrong! Suddenly, I was playing the role of a terror-stricken victim in a horror film! Sheer fear paralyzed me. For those stark, lonely moments, I forgot the Lord.

I quickly returned to my senses and gently reminded myself of the truth: God is not the author of fear. All fear comes from Satan. As a child of God, I shouldn't harbor fear. However, recognizing the source of my fear and affirming God's love did not bring enough relief. Despite my comforting inner dialogue, fear swept over me like wildfire.

I could actually hear the red-hot blood pounding as it rushed through the veins and arteries of my head. Tossing about in bed, I sought a position that would allow me to escape the familiar sounds. In despair, I grasped my aching head between my hands.

Horrible thoughts plagued me throughout the night. I might have an inoperable brain tumor like Helen, my dear friend who died a slow, agonizing death. I could have a stroke and become an invalid for the rest of my life. I'm only in my forties, but Mother was forty-six when she died. That's too young for anyone to die.

I had never allowed myself to entertain such dark thoughts before, but now the terror smothered me like a blanket. I cried and clutched my damp pillow during the long night. Finally, I turned to my only real source of strength and whispered, "Jesus." Of course! "Jesus!" I whispered again. My heart leapt at the sound of His precious name.

I had been lost in a foggy sea where I had forgotten Him for those few, desperate moments. I scolded myself sharply, "How could I have been so careless with my thinking? I've been ministering to people for years on how to 'take every thought captive to the obedience of Christ.' (See 2 Corinthians 10:5.) I must gain control and pull myself out of this depression!"

At that moment, I needed someone who would agree with me in prayer that the Adversary was not going to win this battle. Unfortunately, I had only the emergency number of the Prescott Church Camp, and it would be unthinkable to wake Elmer at 2:00 in the morning. I got out of bed and turned the television dial to a Christian program. For years I had appeared on Christian programming, a veritable "pillar of strength," offering solace and hope to the needy—and now I was on the receiving end at 2:00 A.M., sleepless and shaking!

CBN was playing a rerun of *The 700 Club.* I don't remember who was on or what they were saying. I just waited for the number to appear on the screen so I could dial cross-country, as if that phone wire stretching across the nation was my very lifeline.

The counselor's loving voice brought me immediate comfort. I didn't give her my name. I told her we were missionaries and that I was very sick. More tears flowed as I asked her to pray. But this time they were not tears of self-pity, but tears of gratitude for God's help in my greatest time of need. The counselor graciously offered a few words of encouragement and a short prayer. I thanked her and hung up.

Spying Out the Land

The crisis of this battle had ended, but my fighting had just begun. Although feeling immeasurably better, I decided that the suspense of not knowing exactly what was wrong with me was unbearable. As much as I questioned modern medical technology, I decided to consult a doctor for a diagnosis in the morning.

I really wrestled with that decision. Years ago I had promised myself that I would never go to a medical doctor again. I believed that using drugs to cure an illness only poured in more poison from which the body must recuperate. After all, side effects accompany each medication—and some are worse than the illness itself! Simple logic tells us that we don't get well by taking poison! Still, I wanted to consult a medical doctor. But I vowed to refuse his drugs, no matter what. My prognosis soon tested that vow!

My aversion to the medical profession was for a good reason. From childhood on, I had spent years in a sickbed, mostly in hospitals. Doctors had sedated me several times for various operations and procedures. Once I even had surgery performed on me that turned out to be a complete mistake!

Nevertheless, I decided to seek a professional opinion. Later I would determine how to best proceed. During this long night of turmoil and decision making, my mind turned to the Bible. Before the Israelites entered Canaan, they sent spies ahead to *"view the land"* (Joshua 2:1).

Similarly, I wanted to discover what kind of enemy the Lord and I would be fighting. I didn't expect the doctors to fight for me, only to help me *"spy out the land"* (Numbers 13:16) by locating and naming the problem. Then God would provide me with an effective strategy for my healing.

That evening, I soberly acknowledged that simplistic thinking or swallowing a few aspirin would not alleviate my problem. This was a problem that God and I would handle together. He would guide, and I would obey. We had already discovered half of the solution—prayer. Convinced of God's leading, I knew tomorrow's diagnosis would give me specific information on how to pursue my healing.

A Dire Diagnosis

"You are too young to have this, Mrs. Bueno. This is a disease for the very elderly." Dr. Davis bluntly plunged in with his diagnosis—one that was much worse than I had anticipated. "You have rheumatoid vasculitis, sometimes called temporal arthritis. It affects the entire circulatory system in the body and especially impairs the main artery leading up to the brain. Allergies cause these rheumatoid diseases."

Next, the doctor gave me a page on rheumatoid vasculitis that had been photocopied from a thick medical book. He also handed me a booklet with a grotesque picture of an old lady who was crippled with a rheumatoid disease.

Speaking with a strange mixture of coolness and sympathy that started my adrenaline flowing, Dr. Davis noted, "These materials will explain what you must do to live with this illness. What you have is incurable. At any moment you could suffer a heart attack or stroke, which, if you survived, could precipitate early senility."

I didn't care for Dr. Davis' direct approach, but I appreciated his truthfulness. Perhaps he thought I could cope better if I hit the problem head-on. He advised me to avoid driving, flying, or singing—activities that put added strain and pressure on the arterial system. Finally, he offered me cortisone.

I knew enough about cortisone without having to take it. This highly toxic drug carried horrendous side effects. Many patients experience inordinate weight gain accompanied by a puffy, moon-shaped appearance that distorts all facial characteristics.

"Dr. Davis, I don't like the idea of taking such a powerful drug."

"The cortisone will alleviate your most severe symptoms. But the relief promises to be temporary at best," the doctor admitted. "This disease will always remain in your body."

"What would happen if I decided not to take the cortisone?"

"Frankly, Mrs. Bueno, you will die."

The cold, hard truth frightened me, but at least I knew what was wrong! When it came to treatment, however, I would no longer listen to Dr. Davis. I was even more determined to reject a drug therapy that only masked symptoms and accentuated side effects. Praying for God's guidance, I decided to look elsewhere for treatment.

Before I left Dr. Davis' office, his assistant drew attention to my badly bloodshot eyes. They had looked so red a couple of months previously when we did our last TV taping for *Buenos Amigos,* our weekly Spanish program, that I had asked the cameramen not to take any close-ups. Although I thought that the visit to the dentist somehow related to my present problems, I hadn't even remotely associated the redness of my eyes with the pain in my head—or to Dr. Garcia's treatment.

"Your veins are inflamed and swollen ten to fifteen times their normal size," Dr. Davis' assistant explained. "This prevents the blood from flowing properly. The condition is much like an inebriated man whose veins abnormally constrict from the poisoning effects of alcohol. This inhibits the flow of blood, forcing it to spill over into the eyes. In your case, the inflammation could easily result in blindness."

This sobering statement spurred me on to refuse even an aspirin. As I listened to the doctor's stern warnings, my adrenaline ran rampant and my face flushed. All I knew for sure was that I wanted out of this office! I needed to hear a solution rich with hope and healing, not laden with darkness and doom. I thanked Dr. Davis and his assistant, telling them I was a great believer in proper nutrition, fasting, and even miracles! I left the office and softly closed the door behind me. While walking to my car, I whispered to myself, "If it was a diagnosis I wanted, a diagnosis was what I got!"

On the way home, I stopped to pick up a book I had been intending to add to my home library: *The Pill Book—The Illustrated Guide to the Most Prescribed Drugs in The United States.* I waited until I got to the safety of my home to turn to prednisone, the generic synonym for the doctor's cortisone. As I read, my heart pounded with panic. Once the symptoms of my rheumatoid vasculitis had been masked by this steroid, the remainder of my life would be spent learning to live with its side effects and adverse reactions.

Doctors prescribe prednisone for a variety of disorders from skin rash to cancer. Because of its effect on the adrenal glands, the dosage must be tapered over a period of time. Stopping this medication suddenly or without the advice of a physician could result in the failure of the adrenal glands and serious consequences. Prednisone may mask signs of infection and decrease resistance to new infections. Those taking prednisone should not be vaccinated against infectious diseases because of the body's inability to produce a normal reaction to the vaccine.

A variety of side effects accompany prednisone, including upset stomach, gastric or duodenal ulcers, retention of water, heart failure, potassium loss, muscle weakness, and loss of muscle mass. Loss of calcium may result in bone fractures and the degeneration of the large bones in the hip. Calcium deficiency will also slow down the healing of wounds and bruises. Those taking prednisone may also experience increased sweating, allergic skin rash, itching, convulsions, dizziness, and headaches.

Prednisone may also cause irregular menstrual cycles, hypersensitivity or allergic reactions, blood clots, insomnia, weight gain, increased appetite, nausea, and feelings of ill health. This drug is also known to slow down growth in children, depress the adrenal and pituitary glands, lead to the development of diabetes, and increase fluid pressure inside the eye. This medication may also cause euphoria, mood swings, personality changes, and severe depression. Prednisone may also aggravate existing emotional instability.[1]

Need I say more about my extreme aversion to opting for the drug solution?

Getting a Second Opinion

After my diagnosis, I sought a second opinion, as well as a third and a fourth. These doctors confirmed everything Dr. Davis had said. Three other medical doctors, one of whom was a neurologist, gave me the same medical explanation, offered the same medication, and gave me the same prediction: I would go blind—or die—if I didn't take their drugs. As an afterthought, all three admitted that their drugs were only "a temporary solution."

I remember asking each of the doctors about the dentist's visit and my subsequent head pain. All three insisted the dental work and my pain were not connected. But the still, small voice inside me kept insisting that they were all wrong!

In the face of these well-meaning scare tactics to take the medication, I stood firm, but it wasn't easy. Because society programs us to obey the doctor's orders, it's difficult to follow the Lord's directions, especially when a huge gulf separates the two. I wanted to do what God said, but I had to combat the guilt games most of my loved ones tried to play with me.

Friends and family pressured me to follow the doctor's orders. When I resolved before God that their admonitions would not cause me to waver, some treated me as if I had betrayed them. Some cried. Some got angry. Virtually everyone warned me, "You'll be sorry!"

Because my decision to take "the alternative health care stream" and to bypass "the main medical route" was so out of the ordinary, I suddenly found myself alienated. My husband, son, and daughter were tremendously supportive and in complete agreement with seeking God's natural healing over prescription drugs.

Even my Christian friends found my choice difficult to accept. As a result, when I needed their support most, I was left alone, unable to seek their counsel. These loved ones were just too deeply entrenched in the medical mentality. They also feared that my decision to go against the advice of four "perfectly good doctors" might even be the death of me! Of course, I appreciated their concern, but I had to look for true direction from God.

During this time, the Phillips translation of Romans 12:2 gave me great comfort and courage. *"Don't let the world around you squeeze you into its own* [mold]." I didn't want to be arrogant, belligerent, or foolish, but I had to analyze the whole situation myself. After all, it was my life.

I began talking to myself once again: "This disease has been diagnosed 'incurable.' This may simply mean that the doctors just don't have the answer. If I had broken my leg, it would have been easy. A doctor knows how to set a broken bone, and I wouldn't hesitate to have him do it. But why should I take a drug whose side effects include, among other things, heart failure, while I indulge in only 'temporary relief'? It just doesn't make any sense at all."

Besides the highly recommended cortisone, each doctor had offered me a variety of pills to ease my intensifying pain. I chose not to kill the pain with drugs. I wanted clarity—not oblivion—so that I could be sensitive to changes in my physical state. I especially wanted to note any signs of improvement when the Lord started to heal me. If my body were numbed by the pills, my mind would also be foggy. How would I be able to hear the Lord speaking in that state of semiconsciousness? I had to combat this rheumatoid vasculitis without drugs and with God at my side.

I had spied out the land and identified the problem. Now it was time to pray. "Oh, Lord Jesus, give me the right strategy. Will I march around the walls for seven days, as the Israelites did when they captured Jericho? Or do I charge straight ahead against the enemy?"

Discovering the Healing Formula

Then I remembered my last comment to Dr. Davis upon leaving his office the day of my diagnosis. In an effort to cast out the spirit of "incurable darkness" he had foreseen for me, I had tried to encourage myself by mentioning my faith in nutrition and fasting. Suddenly I knew I had found the other half of my healing formula—fasting!

"Do I *really* believe all that I have learned about fasting?" I asked myself. I had already fasted several times that year and had received healing. After fasting and giving close attention to my health, I was puzzled that such a devastating disease—especially one supposedly caused from an allergy—had incapacitated me.

"If I *really* believe what I've learned about fasting—and I do—then now is my greatest opportunity to prove its validity!" I answered myself. If I believed in the Bible and divine healing, now was the time to become the living example of all those promises. I knew that physical healing and spiritual healing would work hand in hand to cure this so-called incurable disease.

I had never felt so perfectly right on course and so encouraged in the Lord as I did then—the very same moment when the doctors would have me making plans to polish up my coffin!

After this question-and-answer session with myself, I knew what I had to do: find a place where I could safely and comfortably undergo a fast. And that's exactly what I did.

Two

My Healing Fast

Once I determined to fast and pray for my healing, I chose a pleasant spot in northern California. This old farm house, situated in the middle of a walnut grove, had been turned into an eleven-bed complex. I found that it was the perfect refuge for physical and spiritual fasting. The director had created a true sanctuary by not allowing television or newspapers to penetrate the quiet. The staff encouraged the guests to rest with a prescribed two hours of quiet time in the afternoon and an enforced bedtime of 9:30 each evening.

Guests were further cautioned to avoid the energy drains inherent in stimulating conversations and mindless chatter. We were advised to provide the ideal conditions of physical, mental, and spiritual quiet needed so the body could generate sufficient energy to repair and heal itself. During this time, the staff monitored our vital signs, ensuring a professionally supervised fast. After breaking the fast, we gradually began to eat only the best natural foods.

The director had wanted me to fast thirty or forty days or "as long as it takes" for my body to generate enough nerve energy to cleanse itself, providing I had adequate reserves. During this fast I would abstain from ingesting anything but water, rest as much as possible, and be monitored by a trained fasting supervisor.

I certainly had no desire to stay away from my family that long. After all, this would be my third supervised fast away from home in less than a year. Breaking the fast would take two or three weeks longer. Despite the director's drugless prescription, I just couldn't bear the thought of being away from my family that long. "I appreciate your advice. I'll pray about it and see how I progress," I informed him.

During the next several weeks, I thoroughly enjoyed reading Scripture for hours and even whole days! My demanding schedule as an evangelist had never allowed such a luxury in my entire life! My large box of study material included both inspirational reading and health and fasting books. Although the noisy pain in my head never left during the entire fast, I still spent my waking moments pleasantly reading and meditating. Even more important, I spent my time in prayer and fasting, which would soon prove to be an unbeatable combination for total healing.

Being faced with an incurable illness caused me to reevaluate my life during my fasting retreat. The issues that seemed so important just yesterday no longer beckoned for my attention. Many times over the years, I had considered our ministry of television and crusade work too much of a struggle. I had even considered giving it up.

While pondering my present physical condition, I was glad I had persevered. At that very moment, I delighted in not having to rearrange my life to adapt it to what Christ really wanted for me. I was convinced that I was already doing exactly what I would choose to do, even if today were the last day of my life. I determined this as I overlooked the gnawing pain, which I now stoically viewed as my own version of the apostle Paul's *"thorn in the flesh"* (2 Corinthians 12:7). The Lord would remove it in response to my prayer and fasting. I lifted up my sickness to Him and simply waited for my healing.

My Promise from God

The second morning at the sanctuary, I awoke when one of the attendants brought me a fresh pitcher of water. The sun hadn't burned its way through the morning fog yet. I switched on the lamp and reached for my Bible. I asked Helen to heat the water and pour it into the china cup I had brought from home. This was my favorite time of day, sitting propped up in bed with two fluffy pillows, sipping the hot water and pretending it was my morning cup of coffee.

I had brought three translations with me, but this morning I selected *The Living Bible.* Turning to Deuteronomy, I read a series of verses that sprang off the page and into my heart. I allowed them to sink deep into my spirit. I opened the nightstand drawer, took out a pen, and marked four verses. "These are mine," I whispered. God had revealed His plan for my healing. He promised to restore my health and cure the "incurable." It would not happen suddenly, but my healing would come a little at a time.

God explained to the Israelites that they would not inherit the promised land all at once. There were still seven nations they had to conquer. God gave the following instructions to His people:

> *No, do not be afraid of those nations, for the Lord your God is among you, and he is a great and awesome God. He will cast them out a little at a time; he will not do it all at once, for if he did, the wild animals would multiply too quickly and become dangerous. He will do it gradually, and you will move in against those nations and destroy them. He will deliver their kings into your hands, and you will erase their names from the face of the earth. No one will be able to stand against you.* (Deuteronomy 7:21–24 TLB)

This passage confirmed the direction for pursuing my healing. In the same way that the Israelites had the promise of their land, I had the promise of my healing. Like the Israelites, I would not get my promise of healing all at once. God planned to teach me the discipline I would need to keep my healing:

1. I must undergo this period of prayer and fasting.
2. I must learn to adopt an energy-conservative lifestyle.

Like the Israelites who could not receive their promised land all at once, I had to wait for my healing. Understanding this, the fruit of the Holy Spirit—patience—settled in and became my companion.

These key verses in Deuteronomy injected me with the determination I needed. I would move in against the enemy—my illness—and destroy it. That's what the Israelites did. As surely as the kings of the enemy nations had been delivered into the hands of the Israelites to have their names erased *"from the face of the earth,"* my illness had been delivered into my hands. God had handed me the weapons of prayer and fasting, and now He wanted me to use them to erase this incurable illness from my life. I personalized every phrase of this passage. When the pain persisted, I did not allow my faith to waver.

Pain Is a Friend

My symptoms, which were bearable in the beginning of the fast, intensified until constant pain and discomfort prevailed. At this point the director explained a concept quite foreign to our thinking. Fasters should not suppress pain and discomfort with aspirin, prescription drugs, and pills while the body heals itself. The drugless way of healing teaches this concept: pain is a friend. Pain in the body signals the mind about one of two conditions:

1. A problem requires you to alter energy-draining living habits.
2. As a result of changing your energy-draining living habits, bodily healing is going on.

Most Americans have cultivated lifestyles that squander energy, so their pain delivers the first message. At the core of their pleasure-seeking consciousness is the desire to avoid pain as a friend. By turning to painkillers, they deaden nerves that relay life-sustaining messages.

During my supervised fast at the sanctuary, I was not receiving the first message. Because I was fasting, I was receiving the second message. My body was eliminating poisons that had caused the pain. As my body released its toxic overload, my pain increased. This time, however, the elimination—not the buildup—of poisonous waste caused my pain. Like a person with food poisoning who experiences the unpleasantness and pain of vomiting to rid himself of a toxic overload, I was experiencing the unpleasantness and pain of my own self-poisoning. This acute discomfort is not pleasant, but it is necessary to achieve restored health.

Experiencing some unpleasantness in order to get well may sound like twisted logic. While you may feel weak during a fast, your body takes advantage of ideal conditions to repair and heal itself. As a result, your body will put an end to all pain and all disease!

My Healing Crisis

Three weeks passed at the sanctuary, and I decided to break my fast. The next morning, I opened my eyes to find they were badly bloodshot. I couldn't believe it! Fasting for three weeks and now this! Besides that, the location of the pain had dropped from the side to the back of my head. This devastated me! I was drowning in fear once more.

Immediately, I called Elmer, rousing him from his early morning sleep. "Elmer," I agonized, "I woke up this morning with bloodred eyes. They look terrible. You know what that means?" I paused. His silence let me know that he, too, was stunned. "Three long weeks of fasting, and now this! Can you believe it? I know this may sound strange, Elmer, but I've made a decision. Please come and get me right away. I want you to take me to the Stanford University Hospital. I've decided I want a brain scan. I am still sick." I began to cry as the fear drove me to reverse my decision and give up. "This pressure at the back of my head is so unbearable, I can't even sit up, let alone stand on my feet!"

Elmer always stays calm in the midst of a crisis, and he reminded me of God's promises. He prayed over the phone while I listened and silently wept. Then I returned to my bed where I tried to relax and regain my composure. Reaching for my Bible, I opened it to renew my mind and rethink God's promise in Deuteronomy. I meditated on every phrase.

Two hours later, I dialed Elmer's number again. He had been out jogging and praying, as was his usual custom. That morning he had interceded especially for me. I apologized for my earlier panic, explaining that I felt better and he could forget my request for medical intervention. "Naturally, the bloodshot eyes are a great disappointment," I added.

The following day was Sunday. Although I had eaten six small meals in the past two days, I still couldn't stand up. The pressure at the base of my head forced me to lie down. The director reprimanded me sternly for breaking my fast too soon: "You're still detoxifying, and you shouldn't have disturbed that by eating. It's like climbing a ladder. You have to use the same steps coming down that you used going up. Your pain is trying to tell you that you are getting well. Can you remember that pressure-pain near the onset of your illness?" he asked.

I had to think for a moment, and then it came to me. "Yes! That Friday morning, four days after my trip to Tijuana. The pain at the base of my skull felt as if my head was full of infection." I reached up to massage the back of my head. "Yes, it does feel like that same pain." The director assured me that my body had conserved enough vital energy through my fast to release the toxic buildup. My body had undertaken a large scale house-cleaning.

In the language of natural hygiene, this is formally known as a "healing crisis." A healing crisis is the manifestation of a symptom, or group of symptoms, during the body's detoxification and repair. Such crises may be the manifestation of the release into the bloodstream of the morbid, stored by-products of exogenous and endogenous poisoning, producing temporary irritation in various parts of the body. All healing crises, therefore, are simply indications of cleansing processes.

The director assured me that the red, inflamed vessels in my eyes and the pain were both signs that my body was rapidly releasing toxic waste into the bloodstream for elimination. He urged me to be patient. "You're still doing all the right things, so you can only get better. You're resting, sleeping, and conserving energy. You may not be fasting now, but your diet consists of the best energy-conserving foods: fresh, raw fruits and vegetables. Your body is still conducting the detoxifying process."

My discussion with the director shed more light on this principle of symptomatic reversal during fasting, which encouraged me. Miraculously, by the end of the day, my eyes had almost completely cleared, the pressure-pain had disappeared, and I could walk again with no pain in my head! The healing crisis had passed.

My Revelation

Monday morning was my last full day at the sanctuary. The only symptom left was a funny, twitching sensation on the left side of my face. The spasms had started three or four days earlier. After beginning in my lip, they spread to my jaw and the left side of my nose.

I never realized this was a detoxifying symptom. After all the other symptoms had disappeared, I reassured myself that this twitching would leave, too. Through my dedication to prayer and fasting, I had made a faith-inspired comeback from my scare the day before. I refused to allow any lingering symptom to bother me.

The following day, Elmer would arrive to take me home. In my room, I closed the door so as not to disturb anyone else. Even in the midst of all the excitement of feeling so good and seeing Elmer for the first time in weeks, I felt a strong urge to distract myself (or so I thought) by turning on the radio. I automatically turned on a local talk show featuring a dentist from San Francisco.

Little did I know that the Lord was about to provide all the answers on how I had been poisoned into the deadly disease of rheumatoid vasculitis in the first place. And what good timing He had! First, He provided the powerful antidote of prayer and fasting to combat this disease. Second, He ended my stay at the sanctuary with the answer on how and why I had contracted this "incurable" disease.

The first caller confided, "I'm scared to death to go to a dentist ever again. Last year, I went in just to have my teeth cleaned. The next day I was admitted to the hospital with a terrible head infection."

This dentist explained to this woman the cause of her infection. "If the patient has a history of rheumatic fever or a rheumatic heart, the attending dentist should give an antibiotic to prevent infection. He should administer the medication to the patient even before the dental work begins. Probing around in the mouth with sharp instruments, even for the simple process of cleaning, could cause a problem in persons having your special rheumatic history."

The final part of his simple explanation totally captivated my attention: "Furthermore, an infected tooth directs the infection into the head or even into other areas of the body. This infection most often goes straight to the heart and can result in sudden death. Or the infection can lodge in the brain cavity and cause inflammation there."

That was the revelation for which I had been praying! I remembered that day in Tijuana when I sat in the dentist's black leather chair. Dr. Garcia had not asked if I had a history of rheumatic fever. When I was a child, I had spent two years in bed with it. Not knowing this, she failed to protect me with antibiotics before working on that infected tooth. No wonder that pain had felt like my head was filled with infection! Furthermore, the four shots of novocaine were an overdose of a toxic drug that triggered an allergic reaction in my body. As a result, all four doctors diagnosed my condition as "rheumatoid vasculitis."

As my memory reached back to a specific incident in my childhood, the mystery was unveiled. My bout with rheumatic fever had been caused by an allergic reaction to something the dentist had given me. When I had gone for my diagnosis, Dr. Davis had immediately asked, "Are you allergic to anything?"

Now, after having fasted and received my healing, my hand reached for my twitching jaw and lips. "Of course," I cried out loud. "This is the side that had the novocaine!" The novocaine had affected my jaw and the left side of my lips and nose, exactly where the spasms are now taking place! I called for the director to come in immediately. Excited at understanding the cause of my symptoms after months of feeling victimized by a mysterious, "incurable" disease, I told him, "Now I know what caused my illness and why my face is twitching! My body is eliminating the novocaine that has been trapped in there since my visit to the dentist several months ago."

"Do you taste the novocaine?" the director asked. I told him I didn't. He assured me, "Before it's all over, you will actually taste the drug when your body finally releases it."

Sure enough, at 2:00 A.M., the strong, unpleasant taste of chemicals in my mouth awakened me. This symptom lasted until 11:00 A.M. Then the bad taste and the twitching both left. After all those months of pain, my ordeal was finally over. Three long weeks of fasting and four days of eating natural, energy-conserving foods had detoxified me! I had been healed in the name of Jesus.

"That Could Be Me!"

David Maines hosts *100 Huntley Street,* a Canadian Christian television program on which I appeared to share my healing miracle. A few days after my appearance, I received a letter from a woman who wanted to know more details of my healing. Her neighbor had told her of my testimony.

> Dear Lee:
>
> Apparently you had the same problem I now have—temporal arthritis or inflammation of the arteries and blood vessels of the head. It certainly would be helpful to compare notes. Did the Lord heal you? I have been on prednisone for a year, and I can no longer tolerate the side effects. I'm having a secondary infection from the drug right now. I'm especially concerned with losing my eyesight. Can you please help me? This drugging solution is soon to become worse than the disease itself.
>
> —Marjorie

As I sat down to write to Marjorie, my heart melted with compassion. For a moment, I relived that horrible night of terror, helplessness, and pain. That same night led me back to the Lord and to His prayer and fasting antidote.

I felt burdened for all the Marjories who don't have the Lord's antidote available for their immediate use. Doctors' prescriptions and pharmaceutical arsenals are easy to come by, but the simple message of prayer and fasting combined with healthful living practices is hardly known.

Next, the emotion of horror hit me. Just think—that could be me today, addicted to prednisone and suffering from all those side effects and a secondary infection from the drug itself! Marjorie's letter confirmed my belief that prayer and fasting brought healing. God had ministered to me day by day until I was healed.

More than five years have passed since the Lord cured me of an "incurable" disease. And I feel wonderful! My eyes have never again turned bloodshot, nor have the noise and pain ever returned. I feel so good, in fact, that I feel as if I have a born-again body.

My battle with the Enemy in my promised land for health has been won. God and I are the victors. He is the greatest partner anyone could have. His weaponry of prayer and fasting followed by your obedience to His laws of life are unbeatable. Just think of it! He is there for you—right now!

I pray that the truths on prayer and fasting in this book will challenge, encourage, and help you. Please read on with an open mind and an open heart. Even if medical science has pronounced a dire diagnosis over your ailment, you can be helped through the natural means of prayer and fasting.

Three

Launching My Health Ministry

In the days, weeks, and months that followed my healing during the twenty-one day fast at the sanctuary, I began to receive strong urgings from the Lord to expand my ministry from evangelism to health evangelism. God prompted me to search for more knowledge about fasting, superior nutrition, and the other essentials of health and then to share this material as a whole new ministry. I spent the next several months searching for information on fasting so that I could help the sick and suffering choose the drugless, natural route to getting well.

At times my search was frustrating, but also successful. During the next few years, I founded my health ministry, which I named Born Again Body, Incorporated. I amassed the available information and produced a series of audio cassettes, booklets, taped television programs, and this book. I also held several one- and two-week "Genesis 1:29" conferences—named in commemoration of God's original diet proclaimed in the Garden of Eden.

How did I gain the information for my tapes, booklets, and this book? Like a determined gold miner, I persistently chipped past discouragement, dead ends, and frustration before discovering these precious truths. My research, which continues to this day, started several years ago.

My Search Begins

Elmer and I had a real treat on our hands—four days to spend together, just the two of us, doing whatever we pleased in Dallas. Besides just relaxing, I had one special project on our agenda. After lunch we dashed across the busy street in the rain, sharing an umbrella. Opening the heavy glass doors of the Dallas Public Library, I paused and stared at the size of this huge edifice. The impressive array of books fit the Texas reputation for everything coming in the king size.

Not knowing where to begin, we shared our needs with a librarian. "I want to look at books on fasting."

"On what?"

"Fasting."

"Oh, fasting!"

You could read the amazement on her face. I imagined that she would tell friends for weeks about my wanting a book on such a strange topic. To her credit, however, she immediately moved into the role of an efficient librarian. She showed us how to operate the computer to search their resource system for books. While she explained, I wondered why I hadn't thought of using the public library before. I had frequented secular bookstores and health food stores for years, and I had located some material in a few of these specialized places. More often than not, however, my search revealed that little had been written on fasting in the past thirty years.

Exhilaration swept through me as I prepared to use their sophisticated computer. The thought that Dallas' high-tech, computerized library was about to supply me with a long list of reference books and study aids thrilled me! Just think! No more long, draining, wasted hours searching in one health food store after another! I punched in the correct data, and in a split second a short list of books on fasting appeared on the screen in front of me. All were recent titles, and all were available in the United States.

Had I been a gambler in Las Vegas, I might have hollered, "Jackpot!" But I sighed with the relief that comes at the end of a long search and whispered, "Hallelujah!" After jotting down all the code numbers, I began to scan the shelves. My short-lived triumph turned into deep disappointment. The Dallas library did not carry even one of these titles.

After returning to California, I visited several libraries and met the same dead ends. Later I spent several days in the University of California Biomedical Library in Irvine. Their books and journals concentrated on the physical results of fasts conducted with the subject under some sort of medication. The only title that sounded like the type of book I wanted was copyrighted in 1926. Out of desperation, I decided to look at it. Because it was such an old book, however, the library kept it in storage. Procedure required that I put in a request, and they would pull it out of storage by the next day. Upon returning, eager to see what this book might uncover, I learned from the librarian that it was no longer available.

I had bought a few books that approached fasting from the Christian perspective, which recommended other books. So back to the library I went. Even though fasting books by religious publishers may be listed on the computer, they are not readily available in the public library system. One helpful librarian suggested I order them. "But," she cautioned, "since they are out of our jurisdiction, it would take at least two months and perhaps as long as two years. Even then it may be impossible to secure them." Finally, I gave up on the library system.

Perseverance accompanied my new calling as a Christian health missionary, so I continued my search in other ways. After all, I already had the most profound knowledge of fasting available to anyone—firsthand experience that saved my life! I returned to my other sources: books written by natural hygienists that I had purchased at the retreats I had visited. Most of these books focused on the therapeutic fast—a fast taken purely for health reasons—and hardly mentioned the spiritual aspect of fasting. I followed up footnotes and references in those books. I also asked other Christians. After all, the Bible mentions fasting (or its synonyms: mourning, supplication, affliction, and mortification) at least seventy-five times! Christians should know something about this spiritual discipline.

During the past hundred years, not many Christians have written on the subject. Generally speaking, these few books contain excellent material. Like the hygienic writers, however, Christian writers are often one-sided in their approach. They focus on only the spiritual fast, to the exclusion of the therapeutic fast.

"With so little information available on the power of Christian prayer and fasting to bring about physical and spiritual healing," I exclaimed to Elmer, "no wonder fasting rarely occurs to the modern mind!"

Few contemporary authors have been inspired to write on the topic. Is this a result of lack of interest, or possibly no desire to deny ourselves the tempting pleasures of this age? Two hundred years ago, books abounded on fasting, especially when connected with prayer. Today, Jews, Roman Catholics, and members of the Orthodox churches retain some form of fasting in their rules for worship. Most of the other denominations scarcely acknowledge fasting as an aspect in ancient worship and as an element in modern ritual. Modern ritual fasts—abstaining from meat on Fridays during Lent, for example—are seldom an actual fast in the true sense of the word.

The Pharisees and the more devout Jews fasted two days a week, Monday and Thursday (see Luke 18:12), in memory of Moses' ascent and descent of Sinai. In memory of Judas, his conspiracy, and Christ's death, the Christians chose Wednesday and Friday to fast. During biblical times, fasting was almost as commonplace as prayer. Scripture shows that prayer and fasting are similar activities yielding synonymous results. Both open heartfelt lines of communication between God and the individual. During biblical times people practiced fasting before, during, and after a great calamity or crisis. Many fasts recorded in the Bible were of a memorial or commemorative nature.

Why No Healing Fast in Scripture?

Fasts of a spiritual nature occur often throughout both the Old and the New Testaments. Fasts undertaken purely for healing are totally absent from the Bible. We can only speculate why the healing fast is missing. People of biblical times ate more nutritiously, took in more pure air and water, and got more sunshine and exercise than modern Americans. Likewise, they encountered less stress and fewer poisonous chemicals and drugs. They experienced less incidence of chronic, degenerative disease. Without a doubt, people led healthier lives during those days. That alone may account for the lack of emphasis on a healing fast throughout Scripture.

Here's another intriguing piece of speculation on why the healing or therapeutic fast may be absent from Scripture: in biblical times the people may have viewed the spirit and body as being inextricably connected—not distinct and separate as they are now viewed in modern, scientific times.

Even when Old English was evolving from the Germanic, Anglo-Saxon language in what was to become England, the body and soul were still so intimately connected that they had only one root word—*hal*—to mean "health," "whole," and "holy." Those three words were used interchangeably! In short, "to be healthy" also meant "to be whole" and "to be holy."

Did the Bible urge the early Christian to fast so often that physical healing was always assured? Perhaps physical healing was not even mentioned because the spirit and body were so intimately intertwined. Did the early believers just assume that physical health would be renewed with fasting? Since the spiritual reason for fasting was always the foremost, could the physical healing inherent in any fast simply be a foregone conclusion and never deemed important enough to state directly?

Perhaps because the therapeutic fast was automatically a fringe benefit of the spiritual fast, fasting for health was not emphasized in Scripture. The early Christians fasted often, and their holiness, wholeness, and health were virtually guaranteed in this discipline.

The Neglected Discipline

I kept asking questions about fasting. Why has fasting held such a prominent place in many world religions? Even religions of some of the world's most backward nations recognize the physical and nonphysical benefits of a fast. Yet so little is known about fasting for physical and spiritual benefits within the Christian community.

Jesus Christ told His disciples, *"When you fast"* (Matthew 6:16, 17), not "If you fast." Jesus assumed that His followers would fast—and fast regularly! Jesus viewed fasting as a sacred obligation, just as important as prayer! Could one of the open rewards mentioned in that passage be physical healing? Once I understood this dictum, I knew I must pass on its significance to others.

I knew that Jesus had fasted. Still, I found myself asking, "Why did Jesus retreat to the wilderness and undertake a forty-day fast?" Christ did not perform even one miracle before His forty-day fast. What was so important about it? Did Christ expect us to follow His example? The apostle Paul wrote of his personal experiences *"in fastings often"* (2 Corinthians 11:27), making it clear that this was a regular part of his life.

Then why, I pondered, are we so ignorant about fasting today? Does the lack of fasting and prayer in our lives explain the superficiality of the Christian experience for so many of us? Is this lack one reason we're so powerless in the face of adversity?

After all this wondering, I began to question those in the ministry about the importance of fasting. Most simply smiled indulgently at me. They often said things such as, "It's all right to fast a little, but you don't want to do anything that would ruin your health."

I often answered, "God tells us in the Bible to fast. Are you saying that God expects us to do something on a regular basis that would harm our health?" I seldom got satisfactory replies. Although I wanted to engage in earnest dialogue on a topic that could mean healing for millions, many theological leaders merely wanted to give token attention to this "fasting-obsessed woman." I soon realized that most Christians—even ministers—knew little about spiritual fasting and even less about therapeutic fasting.

This was not unlike the medical doctor, who, in his training to heal the sick, learns virtually nothing about nutrition and fasting. "Why do ministers who are so well versed on the Scriptures have so little knowledge regarding fasting?" I asked. "You aren't planning a hunger strike, are you?" one man answered. Another told me, "But I am 'well versed' about fasting. I fast between every meal."

Jesus spent forty days doing something that requires the ultimate in discipline. Can it really be such a joking matter? Believers don't joke about their prayer lives. They would be embarrassed to admit they never tithe or give offerings. Yet a surprising number of Christians not only have never fasted, but they actually seem ignorant of—and even defensive about—the topic of fasting as a Christian responsibility and discipline that can bring untold benefits into their lives.

Then it hit me: God has called me into this health ministry to reach these very kinds of people. In the face of ridicule and indifference, I know the truth that can bring health to their lives. Without appreciating the usefulness of fasting, the uninformed and ill-informed only undervalue the power of this discipline. Those left in darkness have but one recourse—to reject fasting as ineffective and then to point to history when fasting has been abused or fallen into the realm of superstition and folklore.

Because of misinformation and misunderstanding, we've relegated fasting to a practice exclusive to the ancients. This has not been difficult to rationalize, either. The last thing any of us wants is to forgo perhaps the single greatest source of pleasure and sin-free indulgence available today—food!

Unfortunately, Christians in our generation have badly neglected fasting. Not only are they unaware of the spiritual power a believer receives during a fast, but they are also unaware of the miraculous physical benefits fasting offers. The Bible promises that if we Christians fast God's way, our healing will *"spring forth speedily"* (Isaiah 58:8).

Hosea warned the Jews that they were perishing *"for lack of knowledge"* (Hosea 4:6). Like today, most of that needless suffering and untimely death resulted from sheer and willful ignorance. Despite the ignorance, indifference, and even hostility of those whom I had approached in my search for the truth about fasting, I remained relentless. I was convinced that God had revealed the important truth for spiritual strength and physical healing to me.

I had much searching, studying, and synthesizing yet to do. Once prepared, I knew that I had a God-given responsibility to spread this good news. Over the years God has allowed me to see lives gloriously changed as a result of prayer and fasting. Yours may be one of them. Before I share specific instructions on how to fast, let's look into the history of fasting.

Four

How Did Fasting Begin?

Elmer and I were riding in the car of a minister friend from the Southwest. When he learned that we had a keen interest in fasting, he told us he had just conducted his own thirty-day fast. Our ears perked up. Such a rare, lengthy fast piqued our curiosity. We shared our mutual experiences of how hard it is to forgo food. "It certainly is," the pastor agreed. "During my thirty-day fast, I ate only one or two meals a day." To him, that was a fast. I'm sure God accepts what we offer in terms of sacrificing the sensual indulgence in food, whether it be a thirty-day fast or only two meals a day instead of three. But that's not a fast in the strict sense mentioned in the Bible and ancient literature.

This conversation caused me to continue searching for the true meaning of fasting in every sense of the word: biblical, historical, and scientific. First, I wanted the strict denotation of the word itself, so I turned to the *Oxford Dictionary.* The word has its origins in the Old English root word *faestan,* meaning "to hold fast" or "abstain." Fasting means "to abstain from food; especially, to eat sparingly or not at all or abstain from certain foods in observance of a religious duty or as a token of grief." Interestingly enough, even in our everyday dictionary, fasting and religious pursuits were intertwined.

Next I turned to another basic text, *The Jewish Encyclopedia.* Although it's impossible to know for certain where or when or how the practice of fasting was born, this book offered a speculation:

> The origin of fasting is disputed by various critics. Some...are of the opinion that it arose from the custom of providing refreshments for the dead; others...that it was merely a preparation for the eating of the sacrificial meal; others, again...attribute the custom to a desire on the part of the worshippers to humble themselves before their God so as to arouse His sympathy; while still others think that...it originated in the desire of primitive man to bring on at will certain abnormal nervous conditions favorable to those dreams which are supposed to give to the soul direct access to the objective realities of the spiritual world.[1]

An Ancient Discipline

Since ancient times, and probably even throughout prerecorded history, men and women have fasted. Practically every religion on record has either required or encouraged followers to practice some form of fasting. For many centuries, people placed so much emphasis on the religious significance of fasting that whenever anyone gave up eating for a time, onlookers assumed it was done strictly as a religious duty. While I have long since lost the reference, I once read that a tribe in the South Pacific defined a nonreligious person as "one who doesn't believe in God and who doesn't fast." Even though millions around the world have fasted and still do, most Christians, especially in the western hemisphere, know virtually nothing about the topic.

How can we learn more about this ancient discipline? Although never accepted as a valid part of the Bible by most churches, the Apocrypha helps us understand the development of fasting. Scholars believe that most of these books were written about two hundred years before the birth of Christ. Their value lies in what they say about life in their time. These books show that the Jews believed that the practice of fasting existed from the earliest of times. For example:

• According to *The Books of Adam and Eve,* Adam fasted forty days. According to the Slavonic version, he fasted for forty days while Eve fasted forty-four days as penance for their sin in the Garden. (This book may have originated in Hebrew between 20 B.C. and A.D. 70.)

• *The Testament of the Twelve Patriarchs* presents fasting as a way to overcome sin. For the sake of chastity, Joseph fasted during the period when Potiphar's wife attempted to seduce him, before and during his days in prison.

• *The Book of Fasts,* the Babylonian *Ta'anit,* reflects the rabbis' perspective on fasting. The *Ta'anit* has four chapters dealing with special fasts decreed for the community because of drought and other forms of divine visitations, such as pestilence.[2]

• Rabbinic literature warns, "He who eats on the Day of Atonement as much as a big date, as much as the date including its seed and who drinks as much as his saliva is guilty."[3] People who lived in arid climates knew that putting stones in their mouths would activate their saliva glands enough to moisten their lips and keep them from swelling. The Old Testament fasting wouldn't have permitted them even to suck on a date seed!

The Bible mentions fasting on many occasions. Let's examine several incidents that prompted people to undertake fasts.

> *Then Ezra rose up from before the house of God, and went into the chamber of Jehohanan, the son of Eliashib; and when he came there, he ate no bread and drank no water, for he mourned because of the guilt of those from the captivity.*
> (Ezra 10:6)

> *Then Esther told them to reply to Mordecai: "Go, gather all the Jews who are present in Shushan, and fast for me; neither eat nor drink for three days, night or day. My maids and I will fast likewise. And so I will go to the king, which is against the law; and if I perish, I perish!"*
> (Esther 4:15–16)

> *Then Saul arose from the ground, and when his eyes were opened he saw no one. But they led him by the hand and brought him into Damascus. And he was three days without sight, and neither ate nor drank.* (Acts 9:8–9)

This strict fasting was usually for short periods of time, such as from sunup to sundown, from twenty-four hours up to three days in duration. Except for the supernatural fast, such as the forty-day fast of Moses, these total fasts were never more than three days in duration. Many times, as with the Ninevites, penitents included their animals in the fast.

> *Then word came to the king of Nineveh; and he arose from his throne and laid aside his robe, covered himself with sackcloth and sat in ashes. And he caused it to be proclaimed and published throughout Nineveh by the decree of the king and his nobles, saying, "Let neither man nor beast, herd nor flock, taste anything: do not let them eat, or drink water."* (Jonah 3:6–7)

Josephus, a Jewish historian who lived during the first century A.D., mentioned fasting in his writings. He emphasized the Jewish institution of fasting as an act of penance in the atonement for sin or as an act of supplication for deliverance.

Why Did They Fast?

During the great monastic movement, especially from the ninth century through 1500, each of the orders was famous for its stoicism. To follow Christ's example in simplicity and fasting, these religious groups rejected the pleasures of the world. To show their indifference to pain and unpleasantness, the monks prescribed regular periods of fasting as a way to eliminate all selfish, worldly impulses. They publicly cited the reasons for each fast and then instructed the converts on how to conduct the fast.

Rigid enforcement of abstaining from food was the rule of the day. Fasting became synonymous with denial, punishment, and pain. During this period in history, fasting earned a bad reputation that causes people to shun this spiritual discipline even today. Here are other reasons why the monastic orders embraced the practice of fasting:

1. To attain self-mastery, self-understanding, or self-humbling. (See Ezra 8:21; Psalm 69:10–11.)
2. To attain spiritual purity. (See Isaiah 58:5–7.)
3. To atone for sin.
4. To mourn for the dead. (See 1 Samuel 31:13; 2 Samuel 1:12.)
5. To supplicate oneself before God so that He would better hear the plea in times of great stress or calamity. (See Ezra 8:21–23; Nehemiah 1:4–11.)
6. To favorably influence God. (See 2 Samuel 12:16–23.)

Throughout history, people undertook fasts for many different reasons. Most of them carried some religious significance. People viewed fasting in the following ways:

1. As a ritual in preparation for waging a holy war. (See 1 Samuel 14:24.)
2. As a form of repentance. The Ninevites responded to the preaching of Jonah by confessing their sin and petitioning God for mercy. (See Jonah 3:8; Nehemiah 1:4; 9:1–3; Ezra 8:21–23; 1 Samuel 7:6.)
3. As an accompaniment to the exorcism of demons. (See Matthew 17:14–21.)
4. As a penance for fornication. (See 2 Samuel 12:15–16.)
5. As a means to drive out temptation that comes through a full stomach.

6. As a means of self-control. (This practice dates back at least to Plato in 300 B.C.)
7. As a means to end drought. (The *Book of Fasts* in the Talmud contains specific instructions on how to do this.)
8. As a means of strengthening prayer, especially prominent throughout the New Testament. (See Matthew 17:21; Mark 9:17–29; Acts 10:30; 13:2–3; 1 Corinthians 7:5.)
9. As a preparation for baptism in the early church.

In my research I discovered that most of these reasons for fasting fell into five categories:

1. *Purificatory fasting* cleansed oneself from harmful foods. It was also used to purify a youth as he reached adulthood and to purify a woman before she gave birth.
2. *Sympathetic fasting* expressed sympathy for the gravely ill or the dead. (This eventually developed into the practice of fasting during Lent, the weeks that precede Easter.)
3. *Penitential fasting* expressed sorrow for having sinned and often marked genuine repentance.
4. *Meritorious fasting* obtained a reward or secured a level of holiness.
5. *Disciplinary fasting* helped the faster to attain self-control.[4]

Fasting before Christ's Time

References to fasting abound, especially in writings outside of the Old Testament. The Grecian civilization, which flourished before Christ was born, featured fasting as an integral part of their culture. In Jewish theology, the Talmud devotes an entire volume to fasting. It especially emphasized Yom Kippur and the commemorative fast days of the Old Testament era. Other apocryphal writings, especially those in *The Testament of the Twelve Patriarchs* (c. 200 B.C.), make frequent reference to fasting.

Likewise, occurrences of fasting from the same period are found in *The Book of Jubilees. First Enoch* (c. 60–70 B.C.) contains one statement on fasting. Then somewhere near the middle of the first century B.C., *The Psalms of Solomon* appeared with several statements on fasting. Other books you may want to research include the following: *The Book of Fasts,* the Babylonian *Ta'anit*[5]; writings found from the Qumran community; and the works of Josephus, the Jewish historian of the first century A.D. All these texts highly recommend the practice of fasting in specific instances, even though they contain some words of caution.

Except for a few leaders who asked their followers to fast for divine wisdom and a few philosophers who demanded that their students fast for mental clarity, fasting played only a small role in the life of early ancient Greeks.

Later, however, through Oriental influence, fasting became commonplace, especially in the mystery religions such as Kybele, which demanded a partial fast for seven days as an initiation rite. Additionally, those who often gave oracles, such as the prophets and priestesses of Delphi, Patara, Delos, and Claros, claimed that they must first fast as part of their preparation to receive the prophecies. According to legend, these men and women believed that demon forces inhabited certain foods. Those who wanted to contact the gods had to be in a state of ritual purity or they would become contaminated by the demonic.

Another Grecian practice was "incubatio," or sleeping in the temples of certain deities in order to receive prized, prophetic dreams. Greeks considered dreams a key way of making coveted contact with the gods and receiving their divine guidance. In preparation for this practice, Greeks abstained from certain foods known to interfere with sleep. (Beans were on their list!) The participant usually self-imposed a minimum of one day of abstinence from food as an act of self-purification. Others chose to undertake lengthy fasts before "incubatio" as a means to receive dreams with their senses fully sharpened and clear.

Biblical Fasting

Remember the pastor who underwent a thirty-day "fast" and only ate one or two meals a day? The partial fast more appropriately describes his actions. Without any intention of belittling his sacrifice to God, his one or two meals a day contrasts sharply with these ancient fasts, and especially with the prolonged biblical fasts.

To further our study, let us now examine biblical fasting in the strictest sense of the term. The strict biblical fast means one and only one thing: complete and total abstinence from food and water in any of their forms. This is called the total fast, which I'll explain in the next chapter.

Since human life cannot exist much longer than three days on a total fast without supernatural support, this is not the type of fast recommended throughout this book. Unless otherwise specified, I will describe the fast that allows water but not food. This is known as the absolute fast.

By reading just these first few chapters, you should understand that the Christian definition of fasting means much more than the simplistic, intercultural, interfaith definition common throughout history of "abstaining from food and taking only water." Even for the unbeliever, a fast affects his mind, emotions, spirit, and physical body.

But for the Christian, fasting is much more: it is also a physicai exercise to further his spiritual understanding and growth. If the fast is not conducted in such a way as to inspire the Christian to reach out with salvation to suffering humanity, it is a therapeutic fast, with value on the physical plane only.

Remember that Jesus urged His disciples not to imitate the way of the religious leaders of their day. If not eating is the sum of fasting, the Pharisees, in all their pomp and pretense, would have pleased God. After all, they were abstaining from food! Yet the Pharisees flaunted their fasting with a "holier than thou" pretentiousness, lived in direct disobedience, and provoked Jesus into calling them hypocrites.

Do you want to learn how to fast God's way? The next chapter describes several types of fasts and the best times to embark upon them. No matter what your previous experience with fasting, you'll probably find one that's just right for you.

Five

Fasting for All Seasons

Scripture tells us, *"To everything there is a season, a time for every purpose under heaven"* (Ecclesiastes 3:1). God ordained a time for fasting and all kinds of fasts. These fasts fall into three categories: total, absolute, and partial. Along with these three types of fasting, we will also discuss the proclaimed and the individual fasts that are found in Scripture.

What Is a Total Fast?

At a fasting seminar Elmer and I conducted at a church, we discovered that the pastor's wife fasted regularly as she interceded for others. She knew the power in fasting and prayer. She always chose the three-day total fast—no food and no water—when she interceded for someone else.

During one such fast, she prayed for a young man with a drug problem. On the second day of her total fast, her chronic kidney ailment flared up, leaving her too sick to get out of bed. She had previously taken antibiotics for this condition, which had plagued her since childhood. Her doctor had warned that neglecting the medicine would ruin her kidneys. She continued with the fast for the entire three days and refused the antibiotics. Despite such intense pain that she had to remain in bed, she continued to fast and pray for the young man.

After making this decision, she realized that her pain had lessened toward the end of the second day. On the fourth day, she awoke with no pain whatsoever. Miraculously, God answered her prayer for the young drug addict. This woman conferred with her doctor and found that God had completely healed her chronic kidney problem in the process! This woman further testified to us that she has never again experienced another kidney flare-up.

The total fast is conducted by abstaining from both food and water. Some people know this as "the Esther fast," after the example of Queen Esther. (See Esther 4:16.) In modern times, the total fast seldom lasts more than three days. In ancient times, however, longer total fasts are recorded. In the first biblical record of the total fast, Moses completely abstained from food and drink for forty days and forty nights. (See Deuteronomy 9:9, 18, 25–29; 10:10.)

After completing his total fast, Moses started down the mountain, carrying the Ten Commandments written on the tablets of stone. The Israelites had abandoned themselves to all kinds of sinful activity. Outraged by their idolatry, Moses threw the tablets to the ground, and they broke. Turning his back on their paganism, Moses climbed back up the mountain a second time. The Bible tells us that there he fasted another forty days and forty nights.

If not eating for eighty days sounds miraculous, remember that Moses had no water, either. This had to be a supernatural fast because no human can live without water that long. Except for Moses' and Elijah's experiences (see 1 Kings 19:8), other biblical accounts of the total fast were of short duration—usually from twenty-four hours to three days.

Most experts on fasting agree that a total fast should not last more than three days. Even three days is considered risky and is definitely not recommended. We emphasize one rule at our fasting conferences to those who are considering the total fast: go on a total fast only when you know you have received definite and specific instruction from God.

Olga Carroll arrived in Cuernavaca, Mexico, for our first Genesis 1:29 fasting conference in October 1984. After she informed us of her plan to undertake the total fast, we supported her. She had a definite prayer request and felt this was how God wanted her to intercede for a very dear friend. On the third night, exactly seventy-two hours after she had eaten her last meal and drunk her last glass of water, she carried a pitcher of water and an alarm clock into our evening meeting. Olga didn't care about food, but she was thirsty. As soon as the alarm signaled the end of her three-day fast, she was ready to drink!

The Absolute Fast

The absolute fast is a fast in which one abstains from all solid and liquid foods. This fast permits only water, and so some have misnamed it "the water fast." Among fasting experts who use correct terminology, this would be a misnomer because *to fast* means "to abstain." A water fast would mean "to abstain from water."

The absolute fast is also identical with the hygienic fast: it allows only pure water to be taken into the body and encourages as much rest as possible. The absolute fast aids the body in the quickest and most thorough nerve energy restoration, detoxification, and repair possible.

During the total and absolute fasts, the sensation of hunger is absent. Because the body actually feeds on its own reserves, one does not experience hunger. Fasters usually understand this truth: "Appetite is a mental desire; hunger is a bodily need." Since the bodily needs are being met while the body feeds on its available reserves, hunger is absent while fasting. Appetite may be present, but that is not true hunger.

Most theologians agree that Jesus undertook a forty-day absolute fast rather than a total fast—for two reasons. First, the Bible does not specify that He took neither food nor water, as it does in the cases of Moses, Esther, Ezra, and others. Second, Matthew and Luke both said that Christ was hungry after His forty-day fast. (See Matthew 4:2 and Luke 4:2.) Scripture does not say that He was thirsty. Since thirst is a much stronger and more urgent desire than hunger, if Jesus had been without water while fasting, He surely would have wanted it before food.

If you are considering the absolute fast, I offer these suggestions:

1. *Have a phone or office consultation with a professional who understands the benefits of fasting.* Most

of these fasting supervisors will be practitioners of natural hygiene. A listing of these experts can be obtained through my ministry.

Most people can undergo their own absolute fast with nothing but fabulous results. A few people, however (you may be one of them), may need consultation or responsible supervision. A natural hygienist can determine into which group you fall. Although a general rule is to stop all medication while fasting, the immediate cessation of certain kinds of medication can result in death. If you are on no medication at all, however, and if you do not have any of the other contraindications to fasting listed in Appendix 3, you may safely undertake a short absolute fast without the need for this consultation or supervision.

2. *Schedule your absolute fast when you have no demanding physical work.* You need the freedom to rest and sleep as your body requires it. Most people experience weakness. Some people experience restlessness or irritability. These are natural bodily and mental adaptations to fasting. Expect the unexpected. Your body needs to restore and conserve its energy to eliminate toxins and repair its cells, tissues, and organs. When the body's nerve energy is used for work or strenuous exercise rather than for "housecleaning," it is robbed of healing energy, thus slowing the healing and rejuvenation processes.

3. *Fast for one to five days only.* I recommend that you don't enter into an absolute fast for more than five days unless you are an experienced faster or are under professional supervision.

4. *Educate yourself.* Many books and teaching cassettes are available through my ministry that present

more information on the physical and spiritual benefits of fasting. These materials will alleviate your fears about fasting. In fact, they will educate and inspire you to persevere in your time of supplication, prayer, and fasting.

The Partial Fast

To fast means to abstain from something. For example, when we use the term *breakfast,* we mean that we "break the fast" of going without food through the night.

When I explain that I drink only pure water on my fasts, I often get surprised looks from the listeners.

"You mean you don't eat anything?" they commonly ask.

"Yes, and that's why I call it a fast," I reply.

At first I couldn't imagine what they thought when I used the word *fast.* They usually think in terms of the partial fast, whereby I must have taken something, if only vitamin and mineral supplements!

The partial fast means abstinence from certain, select foods and drinks, but not complete abstinence from all foods and drinks. For instance, Daniel abstained from bread, meat, and wine for twenty-one days. (See Daniel 10:3.)

This means that everyone who refrains from eating a particular food is on a partial fast. We do not usually consider vegetarians to be on a partial fast just because they are abstaining from meat. They are practicing a vegetarian eating style, not fasting. Technically speaking, however, they have chosen to abstain from certain foods; they are, therefore, on a partial fast.

People who want to fast but can't stop their medication without suffering dire consequences may want to undertake the partial fast. The body reacts to the sudden withdrawal of certain powerful drugs, such as cortisone, with violent and dangerous results.

A better way to ease off these drugs is to undertake the partial fast with light meals of fruits or with juices. These foods act as a buffer while the toxic cortisone deposits are withdrawn. I recommend that a professional with fasting experience supervise such cases. When people fast for spiritual reasons, I generally suggest that they go on the partial fast to maintain strength so that they can continue their daily routine.

The juice diet is the most popular form of the partial fast. Perhaps the most important items to remember when on the juice diet are to drink fresh juices, consume them slowly, and take no more than five glasses daily.

Just as the uninformed have misnamed the absolute fast "the water fast," they have also given the juice diet the misnomer of "the juice fast." Remember, *to fast* means "to abstain." A juice fast would mean you take in anything but juice! We will use correct terminology at the outset of our study on fasting. Then, if you read some of the more technical writings on fasting, you will not need to relearn the terms used by professionals.

The liquid diet differs from the juice diet because it includes any type of liquid, as long as it is not in the form of a solid food: broth, consommé, hot gelatin, milk, and specially prepared drinks, along with many other beverages. Because many liquid foods available today are not wholesome, I don't recommend the liquid diet for the best physical results. But the liquid diet does sometimes prove a convenient way to fast for spiritual reasons or for weight control.

Daniel's diet was a partial fast. He ate only certain grains, legumes, and vegetables. Since Daniel ate only "pulse," his diet was much stricter than most partial fasts. Pulse includes wheat, barley, rye, dried peas, beans, lentils, and parched corn. According to Scripture, Daniel's diet permitted no animal products such as meat, milk, and eggs. In essence, this is one form of a strict vegetarian diet. (See Daniel 1:12, 16; 2 Samuel 17:28.)

What's the difference between Daniel's partial fast and the Genesis 1:29 diet? Although both are vegetarian, the Genesis 1:29 diet requires no cooking. The person on this diet eats fruits and vegetables in their raw, uncooked state. Because of the types of foods in Daniel's partial fast, they obviously needed to be cooked.

Make a Sacrifice

The partial fast taken for spiritual reasons should eliminate some favorite foods—those we regularly eat—and especially those we enjoy, crave, and overeat. Scripture tells us that Daniel ate *"no pleasant food"* (Daniel 10:3). I believe this means that he ate nothing that excited him or that tasted so good to him that he longed for it. Instead, he ate staple foods, not sensuous foods.

One may use the partial fast to humble himself before God. It can be used as a sacrifice by denying yourself something you like very much. One Jewish man told me that during his days of partial fasting for religious reasons, he gives up his desserts, which he loves dearly.

One of my favorite foods was lobster. Just avoiding it for a month was not a partial fast. Neither is it a partial fast for people who don't like string beans or brussels sprouts to refrain from eating them. Instead, a partial fast is forgoing food that we eat and enjoy regularly.

Here's an example of a partial fast taken for spiritual reasons. My son, Chris, and his wife, Cecilia, fast one day a week. They eliminate sugar, cream, butter, sauces, spices, or any condiments that enhance the flavor of their food. Their meal may consist of fish broiled dry, no butter on the bread, no sugar or cream in the coffee. It's a simple, non-stimulating meal that eliminates the tastiest foods.

I urge people who fast from food to fast from television, newspapers, and hobbies, too. While not technically part of a fast, forgoing the media and other indulgences parallels the discipline needed for the partial fast. This discipline frees time for prayer and Scripture study and helps to remind us that fasting is more than merely going without food.

If the idea of going without any food is not comfortable to you, then the partial fast is a good way to begin acquiring your fasting experience. You do not suffer the physical, emotional, and spiritual shock of having all your food yanked away from you. You won't be left afloat on a sea of foodlessness. After undertaking the partial fast of your choice a few times, you'll learn that you don't need to fear undertaking the absolute fast for a day.

The Proclaimed Fast

After discovering a plot to kill her people, Queen Esther sent a message to Mordecai, saying, *"Go, gather all the Jews who are present in Shushan, and fast for me; neither eat nor drink for three days, night or day. My maids and I will fast likewise"* (Esther 4:16). Such a declaration is called the proclaimed fast.

Have you ever agreed with others in prayer for spiritual strength and guidance from the Lord? Joining others in the proclaimed fast is similar. The proclaimed fast occurs when two or more persons decide to abstain from food for spiritual reasons. They are in agreement in fasting and prayer. The proclaimed fast has also been called the corporate fast, since two or more people join as a single body for a common cause. (*Corpus* means "body" in Latin.)

How were corporate fasts proclaimed in the Bible? A person in authority, such as an Old Testament prophet or king, publicly called his city or nation to fast. Here are some examples from Scripture:

• Ezra proclaimed a fast at the river Ahava so that the Jews could humble themselves before God and seek His direction on their journey to Jerusalem. (See Ezra 8:21–23, 31–32.)

• When the inhabitants of Jabesh Gilead heard that Saul and his sons were slain in battle, they burned the bodies, buried the bones, and fasted for seven days. (See 1 Samuel 31:11, 13.)

• Hearing that three armies had mustered themselves against the Israelites, *"Jehoshaphat feared, and set himself to seek the* L*ORD, and proclaimed a fast throughout all Judah"* (2 Chronicles 20:3).

• As Saul pursued the Philistines in battle, he uttered a rash oath: *"Cursed is the man who eats any food until evening, before I have taken vengeance on my enemies"* (1 Samuel 14:24).

• In a scheme to seize Naboth's vineyard, Jezebel wrote letters in Ahab's name, saying, *"Proclaim a fast, and seat Naboth with high honor among the people; and seat two men, scoundrels, before him to bear witness against him, saying, 'You have blasphemed God and the king! Then take him out, and stone him, that he may die'"* (1 Kings 21:9–10).

These last two examples show that even proclaimed fasts—like some of our personal fasts—were not always done with the best of motives.

In Bible times, leaders often proclaimed a fast so that the people could call upon God for support in overcoming a serious problem, such as a plague or an advancing army. Leaders in the church at Antioch declared a fast to seek the Lord. This resulted in commissioning Paul and Barnabas as the church's first missionaries. (See Acts 13:1–3.)

In the first century A.D., people often fasted before appointing their elders. It seems they didn't fast so that they would know whom to choose as much as to focus on the importance of the event and to sanctify the memorable occasion. (See Acts 14:23; Exodus 34:2, 28; Deuteronomy 9:9, 18.) Their fast also demonstrated to God their willingness to *"afflict their souls."* (See Leviticus 16:29.)

The law of Moses proclaimed only one fast a year on the Day of Atonement. (See Leviticus 16:29–34; 23:26–32; Numbers 29:7–11.) On that day everyone joined as one body to "afflict their souls" in prayer and fasting. According to Julius H. Greenstone, Jewish fasts

> begin at sunrise and end with the appearance of the first star of the evening, except those of the Day of Atonement and of the Ninth of Ab, which last "from even till even."[1]

Laws made provision for young children to undergo some measure of fasting (partial fasting) so that when they grew up, they would be prepared to participate in the national fast. The Bible records other occurrences of the call to a national fast. (See 1 Samuel 20:32–34; Isaiah 58:3–7; Jeremiah 36:1–9; Jonah 3:7–9; Esther 4:16.)

The proclaimed fast didn't end in Bible times. The pages of history describe specific times when people and nations undertook the proclaimed fast at the direction of their leaders:

• For the past 1300 years, strict Muslims have obeyed the proclamation to fast for the thirty days they call Ramadan, during which time they refuse food from sunrise to sunset.

• When the Great Plague struck London in 1563, the king proclaimed a fast until the epidemic abated.

• Throughout the 1600s in England, the Dissenters gained control of the House of Commons and regularly proclaimed fasts. Later, during the period of the

Restoration, the king proclaimed occasional public fasts.

• Before leaving for the New World in the late 1500s, the Puritans held three formal periods of fasting. First, in Holland where they had taken refuge, the leaders proclaimed a fast to seek God's guidance. Second, once they believed they had God's guidance to emigrate to the New World, the leaders proclaimed a fast to commemorate their approaching departure. Third, in a final farewell to England, the clergy proclaimed a fast.

• During the American Revolution, the Continental Congress proclaimed that all Americans should observe July 20, 1775, as a national day of fasting and prayer as they readied themselves for a war of independence.

• Clergy in the southern states proclaimed a fast for November 21, 1860, shortly before the outbreak of the Civil War. The following year, clergy in the North followed suit and proclaimed September 26, 1861, as a day of fasting.

Today, a pastor might formally declare a time of prayer and fasting for his congregation. The proclamation could be for total, absolute, or partial fasting. And it could be for one meal's duration or much longer. Agreement among the fasters sets the proclaimed fast in motion.

The Individual Fast

The individual fast, sometimes called the personal fast, simply means that one person fasts, rather than two or more. Someone may undertake the individual fast primarily for therapeutic reasons. At other times, however, the individual may be led to fast as a religious exercise or during a time of spiritual hunger. Here are some biblical examples of people who undertook personal fasts:

• Hannah grieved over her inability to bear children. Her rival provoked her, therefore *"she wept and did not eat"* (1 Samuel 1:7).

• Ahab, after Naboth refused to sell him his vineyard, *"lay down on his bed, and turned away his face, and would eat no food"* (1 Kings 21:4).

• Anna, an elderly widow who saw Jesus presented in the temple, *"served God with fastings and prayers night and day"* (Luke 2:37).

• Saul, confronted by Jesus on the road to Damascus, *"was three days without sight, and neither ate nor drank"* (Acts 9:9).

• Cornelius, explaining his angelic visitation to Simon Peter, said, *"Four days ago I was fasting until this hour"* (Acts 10:30).

Many spiritual needs can lead a person to fast unto the Lord. (See 2 Samuel 12:20–23; Daniel 6:18; 9:3; Nehemiah 1:4.) People often fast during times of great distress. Let's look at one example in detail.

Evil men encouraged King Darius to sign a decree that for thirty days, whoever petitioned any god or man, except the king, would be cast into a den of lions. Daniel's enemies reported to the king that he violated the law by praying to God three times a day. The king *"was greatly displeased with himself, and set his heart on Daniel to deliver him; and he labored till the going down of the sun to deliver him"* (Daniel 6:14). But because of the signed decree, the king had no choice but to throw Daniel into the lions' den.

> *So the king gave the command, and they brought Daniel and cast him into the den of lions. But the king spoke, saying to Daniel, "Your God, whom you serve continually, He will deliver you."...Now the king went to his palace and spent the night* ***fasting****; and no musicians were brought before him. Also* ***his sleep went from him.*** *Then the king arose very early in the morning and went in haste to the den of lions. And when he came to the den, he cried out with a lamenting voice to Daniel. The king spoke, saying to Daniel, "Daniel, servant of the living God, has your God, whom you serve continually, been able to deliver you from the lions?" Then Daniel said to the king, "...My God sent His angel and shut the lions' mouths, so that they have not hurt me, because I was found innocent before Him; and also, O king, I have done no wrong before you."*
>
> (Daniel 6:16, 18–22, emphasis added)

Afflicting, Humbling, and Fasting

Proclaimed and individual fasts occur in the Bible, usually connected with the idea of afflicting or humbling the soul. (See Leviticus 16:29.) In time, the words *fast* and *to afflict your soul* became interchangeable. As proof of the similarity of *fasting* and *afflicting,* consider the following Scriptures where the writers combine the two terms for emphasis:

> *"Why have we fasted," they say, "and You have not seen? Why have we afflicted our souls, and You take no notice?"* (Isaiah 58:3)

> *Is it a fast that I have chosen, a day for a man to afflict his soul?* (Isaiah 58:5)

> *I humbled myself with fasting.* (Psalm 35:13)

This is the essence of the spiritual fast: to strengthen true repentance and to offer true humility. Such spiritual fasting helps to remind us of our unworthiness as sinners, and it leads us—sometimes in a sense of desperation—to ask for God's tender mercies and forgiveness. Whether practiced by a corporate body in a proclaimed fast or by one person in the individual fast, the fast of repentance and humility is the true spiritual fast. The early Mosaic expression for fasting is "to afflict (bow, humble) the soul" by restraining the earthly appetites that have their seat in the soul.[2]

Pick the Proper Time to Fast

Once you're convinced of the benefits of fasting, you should decide the proper time to undertake a fast. A short fast of one to three days can be taken virtually anytime. Fasting from Friday evening to Monday morning would give you the entire weekend to rest and spend time reading Scripture.

Another ideal time is during vacations from work. You can plan an extended period of several days to fast. You might fast at home, or you may choose to be supervised by an experienced natural hygienist.

The holiday season of Thanksgiving, Christmas, and New Year's may be the ideal time for you to fast. It depends on your own calling, resolve, and time schedule. Generally, I discourage people from fasting during these holidays. With family and friends dropping in and bringing gifts of food, fasting around the holidays is difficult—not only on yourself, but also on others around you.

Be sure to choose an appropriate time to fast. According to your schedule and the various holidays and holy days, certain times of the year will yield themselves as the best times for you to consider fasting for physical and spiritual renewal. The six weeks of Lent, from Ash Wednesday to Easter, are an excellent fasting time.

John the Baptist's disciples and the Pharisees fasted regularly. They noticed, however, that Jesus' followers did not observe special fast days. They asked why. Jesus replied, *"Can the friends of the bridegroom mourn as long as the bridegroom is with them?"* (Matthew 14:17). Jesus had only a short time left with His disciples. This was a time of celebration and fellowship that often revolved around food.

Fasting during the holidays is not wrong. Some people deliberately choose the week between Christmas and New Year's Day to fast. But if the entire family is celebrating, wouldn't it be better to join them in celebration and fast at a more convenient time? God wants His people to feast and to fast. We can be sensitive about the timing of both. The Bible reminds us: *"To everything there is a season, a time for every purpose under heaven"* (Ecclesiastes 3:1).

As the title of this chapter suggests, there is a time for fasting—and there are all kinds of fasts. Be sensitive to fast in God's timing. Simply pray for God's direction on when your season is near—and obey.

Six

Fasting versus Starvation

Bobby Sands, age twenty-seven, died on May 5, 1981, on the sixty-sixth day of his so-called "political fast." He failed to force the British government to grant special political status to him and seven hundred other imprisoned members of the Irish Republican Army (IRA). He did manage, however, to fan the flames of Republican passions and incite street violence to levels previously unseen in Northern Ireland in nearly a decade. Ironically, the results of Bobby Sands' political fast only tightened the tension between the two opponents, the British government and the IRA. Unfortunately, Bobby Sands lost both his life and his battle for his government.

A few months later, Mitchell Snyder, a thirty-eight-year-old Catholic and Christian activist, proclaimed a political fast. Snyder protested against the United States government naming a submarine *Corpus Christi,* Latin for "the body of Christ." Snyder felt the government's decision to put such a name on a warship was sacrilegious. The U.S. government stated it was simply named after the Texan city. Snyder persevered sixty-four days on an absolute fast. The government, wanting to avoid the bad publicity of a Christian martyr going up against them, renamed the submarine *City of Corpus Christi.* Snyder celebrated his victory by sipping a bowl of soup.

Why did Bobby Sands die and Mitchell Snyder live after fasting almost the same number of days? The answer lies in the physiological laws of human life. Everybody is different, and everybody has different amounts of fat, protein, vitamin, and mineral reserves in their tissues. Everybody has differing nerve energy reserves.

Bobby Sands used up these reserves and passed from fasting into starvation. Sands' physiological condition turned into irreversible starvation several days before he died. He willingly ignored his body's signals and chose to commit suicide by starvation. Mitchell Snyder had not used up his reserves and was still in the fasting state when he broke his fast. Accordingly, Snyder still looked healthy when he broke his fast and could have gone on longer.

Most people don't understand the relationship between fasting and starvation. The gaunt faces and emaciated bodies of starving concentration camp victims may still be stuck in your mind. These images may keep you from stepping out on your newfound knowledge and your faith in the Lord.

When does abstention from food and deep rest change from fasting to starvation? When does abstinence become suicide? When does the body signal, "Enough! Stop, or I die!" For people who have never fasted or who have fasted for only one or two days, these may sound like confusing questions. Yet once we understand the principles in fasting and starvation, we have clear answers to these questions. Let's eliminate the confusion once and for all.

Principles of Fasting

After the first two or three days of a fast, hunger leaves. This doesn't mean it's impossible to eat if food were set before us or that the thought of food is suddenly unappealing, but the craving for food disappears. Remember that appetite is a mental desire; hunger is a bodily need.

For example, when I fasted at the Shangri-La in Florida for a physical problem, I heard the menu described in detail from guests who were eating. Fasters at the spas and institutions often gathered to chat. They discussed food, recipes, and restaurants. Even though I listened to and participated in the conversation, their graphic, even mouth-watering descriptions didn't make me want to eat. I was fasting, and I simply was not hungry.

Even when the fifteenth day of my fast arrived, my body was still in the fasting mode, and I simply was not hungry. I felt terrific and wanted to continue several more days. Unfortunately, my schedule wouldn't permit it.

When hunger reappears, it's definitely time to end the fast. Scripture illustrates this principle at the conclusion of Jesus' forty-day fast. *"When He had fasted forty days and forty nights, afterward He was hungry"* (Matthew 4:2). His hunger signaled that He had finished fasting. He had completed his fast.

After we cut off our food supply, our bodies burn fuel reserves stored in the bodily tissues and fluids and simultaneously break down toxic deposits throughout the body. Between the second and third days of a fast, a series of profound biochemical and physiological changes occur in the body. These temporary changes reverse themselves when we begin to eat again. Here are some of these changes:

• *Foul breath, the first sign of detoxification, occurs.* Seventy percent of bodily elimination comes through the lungs. The "gorilla breath" that most people experience upon awakening each morning occurs because the body has been on a mini-fast since its last meal. The body goes into an elimination cycle, and the detoxification process begins.

• *A coated tongue appears.* This shows the accumulation of toxins throughout the thirty-foot alimentary canal that starts at the tip of the tongue and runs through the entire body, ending at the anus. This is another normal area of elimination, as the toxins accumulate in the mucous membranes of the alimentary tract for excretion.

At times, this mucosal accumulation causes the tongue to appear completely white, sometimes even green, thick, and almost furry. The coated tongue will change according to how many days you have fasted or what your diet has been. To the trained doctor, the condition of the tongue gives an accurate reading about the true state of one's health, vitality, and rate of detoxification. Because of the ability of the tongue to reflect the internal condition of the body, the tongue has often been called "the magic mirror."

Medical doctors realize that a coated tongue reveals your state of health and disease. This is why they routinely say, "Stick out your tongue, and say, 'Ah.'" Upon finding a coated tongue, they know that something is happening throughout your system. Few of them with conventional training, however, make any connection between fasting, detoxification, and getting well. Upon spying a white tongue, the first thing they think is, "Disease!" Next, they usually write out a prescription for drugs. Unfortunately, the ingestion of drugs may stop whatever toxic elimination the body had initiated in its attempt to get well.

• *Foul body odors occur.* The largest organ of elimination in the human body is the skin. Its millions of pores allow the toxins to escape. During a fast, the detoxification is often so greatly accelerated that the body takes on unpleasant odors as the poisons diffuse into the atmosphere.

Although momentarily unpleasant, such odors are no cause for alarm. In no way should this odor be associated with the smell of death so often noticed around very sick people who continue to poison themselves with many drugs. The odor of a faster is the not-so-sweet smell of a person getting well!

• *Weakness may occur.* By the third to fifth day of an absolute fast, hunger almost invariably leaves. The body no longer receives food for survival but feeds on its reserves.

Because the body needs a tremendous amount of energy for such profound housecleaning, the faster almost always experiences weakness. Some feel irritable or restless along with the weakness. Take these bodily, mental, and emotional symptoms in stride, knowing that fasting and prayer is the most powerful healing, restoring, regenerating activity you could possibly undertake.

Assuming the faster has enough reserves and nerve energy to take a complete fast, when the body is fully detoxified, then the tongue clears, the breath sweetens, the skin exudes a pleasant smell, and hunger returns. At this point, the fast is ended.

When hunger returns, we must take food immediately. This is where fasting and starvation meet. If food is not taken at this point, the body starts feeding off its essential tissues and not from its reserves. When the body needs its own vital organs for survival, that's true starvation.

We must not confuse fasting with starvation. Unfortunately, the two words are used interchangeably in virtually all medical circles. All but one in a thousand doctors react negatively to the subject of fasting. They have never fasted, know little about the subject, and respond only to bizarre stories that they've heard. Lack of understanding creates unnecessary fear and results in unfounded, imaginary dangers and the use of scare tactics by doctors to avoid fasting.

Remember, fasting is not starving. Fasting begins with the omission of the food, and it ends with the return of natural hunger. In contrast, starvation begins with the return of natural hunger, and it ends with death.

Insight into Jesus' Temptation

Although the Bible doesn't give the physical details of Jesus' fast, it appears that He also conducted the completed fast. After forty days of fasting, Jesus hungered. (See Matthew 4:2.) His body signaled that His reserves were gone and His fast was completed. It was time to take food.

As we learned earlier, fasters do not experience hunger after the first few days of a fast. The return of hunger is a safeguard to prevent starvation. If someone ignores his hunger at this time, the body begins to feed upon its vital organs to survive. This is the first stage of starvation.

This makes the first temptation of Christ even more significant. Jesus hungered; His fast was completed. There were no more reserves left in His body. It was vital to His physical health that He eat immediately to prevent the first stages of starvation.

The temptation to turn stones into bread was more than a temptation to perform what could have been His very first miracle. Taking food was vital to His very life. Christ knew His immediate physical need—and so did Satan. Jesus certainly had more than one reason to yield to temptation.

What did Jesus do? He quoted the Scripture, *"Man shall not live by bread alone, but by every word that proceeds from the mouth of God"* (Matthew 4:4). He trusted His heavenly Father to care for His physical needs. When Satan finished his last temptation, God sent angels to minister to Jesus. (See Matthew 4:11.) I believe that the angels brought Him food.

"How Long Should I Fast?"

People sometimes ask, "How many days will I be able to fast?" No one can determine ahead of time how long a completed fast will take. The seven determining factors are as follows:

1. The available nerve energy reserves
2. The amount of reserves in the bodily fluids and tissues
3. The inherited predisposition of the individual
4. The bodily injuries and traumas sustained in life
5. The degree of toxic buildup present in the body
6. The type of toxic buildup in the body
7. The determination of the individual

These seven determining factors vary widely with each individual. Even a very thin person has days, if not weeks, of reserves. For most of us, it is surprising how long it takes to complete a fast. Completion often occurs around the fortieth day. This, of course, will also vary.

The shortest recorded complete fast was that of Dr. Henry S. Tanner's wife. Dr. Tanner conducted many long fasts of his own that were headline news around the world at the turn of the century. His wife's hunger returned after only ten days.

One very long fast was supervised by Dr. Alex Burton, a fasting expert from Australia. In 1982, Dr. Burton supervised the fast of a man for 103 days. The longest recorded fast is said to have been 365 days. The late Dr. Allan Cott, an expert in the field and the author of *The Ultimate Diet,* stated that he has not known anyone who has truly completed a fast in less than twenty-eight days. These statistics prove that the average person shouldn't worry about starvation if he undertakes short fasts of just a few days.

I've undertaken many fasts in some of the fasting spas and hygienic institutions across the nation. At such places, experts instruct their clients that if their hunger returns while they're on a long fast, even during the night, they need to take nourishment immediately. The director usually says, "If those hunger pains start, immediately knock on my door. I'll escort you to the kitchen for food right away."

A guest at one of these retreats had just started to fast for the first time. After forty-eight hours, he banged on the director's door in the middle of the night, insisting his hunger had returned and that he had to eat immediately.

The director raised his eyebrows and chuckled as he related this story during a lecture. He told his hungry guest, "Go back to bed. You've only been fasting forty-eight hours."

"But my hunger has returned," the man insisted.

"Your hunger hasn't returned," he said, "because it hasn't even left yet!"

Benefits of Fasting

The late Dr. Herbert Shelton, the world's most renowned natural hygiene practitioner of the twentieth century, placed thc following stamp of approval on the practice of fasting: "Fasting is the best way to maintain good health, eliminate pain and disease, reduce and control weight, and ultimately prolong life."

Those who have studied the fasting process attest to its benefits. In no way can it be compared to the life-threatening effects of starvation. Fasting is a normal, biological process for all living creatures. Observe the animals. When dogs or cats get sick or injured, they find a quiet, warm, preferably secluded spot and fast until they feel better. Even their water intake is minimal.

Wounded elephants will continue to travel with the rest of the herd. While the others eat up to two thousand pounds of grass a day, the sick elephants spend most of the time supporting their weight against a tree, sometimes kneeling on the ground, but never eating while sick. They have unerring instincts for the restoration of their bodies. Fasting restores health—it doesn't rob you of health!

In human beings the same rule applies if we pay attention to our bodies. When an acute disease strikes, we tend to lose our desire for food. When we have a cold or the flu, we sometimes complain that nothing tastes good. That's the body's message to us to withhold food from ourselves.

When we lose our appetites, our organic instincts know that to eat in the usual way increases the disease. In our culture, we think the loss of appetite is a great calamity and seek ways to restore it. If we ate no food during these times of no appetite, however, and only minimal food in times of chronic disease, we would:

1. Recover more speedily
2. Avoid a lot of physical suffering
3. Be more in tune with our bodies
4. Possibly lengthen our lives

Dr. Isaac Jennings, a strong Christian man who was posthumously named "The Father of Natural Hygiene" and who was a great advocate of fasting, stated, "It is of no advantage to urge food upon the stomach when there is no digestive power to work it up." Many times the digestive juices stop flowing when there is acute disease. Emotional stress can further cause the outlet of the stomach to contract so tightly that nothing can leave it. This forces the food to sit inside the warm stomach to ferment and putrefy.

Because fasting is the best, natural way to allow your body to heal, it is also the safest way. Fasting makes more sense than eating while you're sick. Unfortunately, engraved in most of our minds is the idea that we must eat "to keep our strength" no matter how we feel about food at the moment. We ignore the quiet language of the body. Fearful of starvation, we compound the crime by force-feeding ourselves and our loved ones. Wanting to avoid emotional scenes by anxiety-ridden family members, we give in and eat. The next time we're sick and have no appetite, we should eliminate mother's chicken soup and follow our natural instincts not to eat until the symptoms subside. Even animals have better sense than we do! We must trust our bodies and admit that God who created them is smarter than we are.

Dr. Hereward Carrington, a member of the Council of the American Institute for Scientific Research at the turn of the twentieth century, gave us an idea of the rejuvenating effect of fasting:

> The moment the last morsel of food is digested and the stomach is emptied, a reconstruction process begins. New cells replace the broken down cells. The replacement of cells means replacement of tissue. The common custom of eating three to six times a day doesn't give the burdened stomach a chance to empty itself so that the repairing of the worn and wasted cells can begin. During a fast, the good cells

> reduce in size. This rejuvenating process begins only after the stomach is emptied.[1]

Seventy-five trillion cells make up each of our bodies. These cells constantly rebuild organs by replacing the old cells with new ones. Dr. Carrington continued:

> This amazing replacement of cells means replacement of tissue; replacement of tissue means a new stomach has been constructed—a stomach new in every sense of the word, as new in every anatomical sense as in the filling in of wounds, or between the fractured ends of bones.[2]

Scientists tell us that the creative force of the human organism is so great that we get a new body every eleven months! Except for the cells in the brain and a few other select places in the body, every one of our 75,000,000,000,000 (75 trillion) cells in the body is replaced so that no organ is more than a year old.

If we're getting new bodies at the cellular level every year, then why are Americans so unhealthy? Because we poison ourselves faster than we detoxify. We don't practice energy conservation in our lifestyles, and we accumulate more toxic waste than we can eliminate through our unhealthful living habits. We defile the temple of the Holy Spirit instead of cleansing it. (See 1 Corinthians 3:16–17; 6:19.)

This book will teach you how to cleanse your body, His temple. We should consider it a privilege to follow our Lord's example in prayer, fasting, and healthful living practices. Most of us have sought instruction on how to pray and read the Bible. We also need instructions on how to fast. Like any other serious and highly useful practice, fasting should not be toyed with or entered into lightly.

When people tell me that they are reluctant to fast or fear harmful side-effects, I remind them that God never expects us to do anything that would harm our health. And He never asks us to do anything that is beyond our capabilities. God does not expect us to starve, but He does expect us to fast!

Seven

The Therapeutic Fast

The therapeutic fast yields tremendous physical benefits through the partial fast, or, more effectively through the absolute fast. If a person has a troublesome ailment and would like to undertake an extended therapeutic fast, his decision would depend on time and money available for a lengthy supervised fast and the seven determining factors listed in the previous chapter. If the goal is to get well as soon as possible, the absolute fast is the first fast to consider.

In a paper called "The Fasting Cure," Dr. J. H. Kellog drew a parallel between a furnace and the human body during a fast. He pointed out that when we don't have our regular meals, we begin to feed upon our stored reserves and bodily wastes. After a day or two, we no longer feel hungry. The body recognizes that it cannot get food, so it burns nonessential tissue to keep going. The body draws from its stored resources and uses every particle of fat, reserve protein, vitamin and mineral excesses, morbid tissue, and superfluous fluids. It also uses only partially digested food.[1]

Dr. Kellog claimed that uric acid, a highly poisonous by-product of protein metabolism, makes up the bodily cinders in his parallel. Our bodies can profitably consume only an ounce and a half of protein a day. A diet containing more than this amount leaves such an accumulation of toxic uric acid ash residue that the body cannot eliminate all of it. These poisons get stored in out-of-the-way places in the body and cause havoc in the form of acute and chronic disease.

On the standard American diet, most people ordinarily eat not the ounce and a half of protein a day, but from three to five ounces per day. The health and nutrition books that support the standard American diet tell people to consume at least three or four ounces of protein daily in order to maintain their health and strength. Army rations supply an excessive four to five ounces. Still, scientific study reveals that a modest ounce and a half of protein a day is all the body should consume to avoid the acid ash buildup.

This means that most of us eat two or three times as much protein as we need. Because we cannot use or eliminate all the toxic acid residue from protein metabolism, it builds up in our bodies as half-burned ashes—like cinders that collect in a furnace until no air can get through the grate. We have to remove the ashes before we can get a bright fire burning.

Dr. Kellog emphasized one significant benefit of fasting: it gets rid of the cinders—the uric acid, or the protein waste of the body. Fasting clears out the acid ash residue and breaks down and neutralizes other waste tissues and deposits. The body always uses unhealthy tissues and reserve tissues before it consumes the vital and essential tissues.

In the completed fast, our bodies eventually lose their morbid tissue. When only healthy tissue remains, hunger returns. The fast is ended. The body has restored itself to health. This is the only cure possible, and it can only be achieved by the body itself.

Tumors Disappear

A high correlation exists between a diet rich in meat and other animal products and the incidence of cancer and tumors among Americans. Standard medical treatment for getting rid of tumors is drastic: it ranges from surgery to chemotherapy to radiation. The success rate is discouraging, and the cost is exorbitant. But the shrinking and disappearance of tumors is simply an automatic fringe benefit among tumor-ridden fasters. And the daily cost at a fasting retreat is less than one-tenth the total daily cost at a hospital.

Many years ago I read about tumors dissolving during a water fast from an explanation given by Dr. John H. Tilden.[2] Dr. Tilden, the world's most knowledgeable natural hygienist during the first half of the twentieth century, was also a strong Christian. Dr. Tilden's landmark book explains that the one cause of all disease is toxic saturation of the fluids and tissues of the body. Since learning that tumors dissolve during a fast, I have witnessed this truth on many occasions. Here are just five examples I have encountered.

At Lake Worth, Florida, in July 1984, a Jewish couple spoke with me after the morning service. Mrs. Albin said, "I went on a twenty-four day fast and dissolved a tumor larger than a grapefruit." These two beautiful people didn't look over sixty-five and enjoyed magnificent health. Mrs. Albin was seventy-nine, and her husband was eighty-five! She told me that they live almost exclusively on fruits and vegetables.

My friend Hilda Warren underwent surgery for breast and lymph node cancer in February 1986. She found a doctor who consented to a lumpectomy rather than a complete mastectomy. Unfortunately, the surgeon missed one of the lumps in her right breast. When she discovered this lump, she was urged to have it removed immediately. First, however, she attended one of our ten-day fasting and prayer health conferences. I supervised a partial fast for her in which she ate uncooked fruits and vegetables and drank fresh juices three times a day. After returning home, she went to the doctor to make arrangements for the surgery. The cancerous tumor was gone!

Doris Pakos, of Glendale, Arizona, editor of *Sweetwater Magazine,* wrote to me on March 20, 1985, after fasting at one of our conferences:

> Dear Lee:
>
> As the conference began you promised that we would never be the same again! That was certainly true. I knew when I arrived at the conference that I had uterine fibroid tumors. They have practically disappeared at this time. I had to have an ultrasound to convince my M.D., so that is now a fact.
>
> —Doris

In my own case, polyps or small tumors in the nose had bothered me for years. They disappeared during a three-week fast. Likewise, a mole on my face that doctors had tried to remove with an electric needle when I was a teenager also disappeared on the same fast.

For over thirty years, my husband had an unsightly growth on his back that was about the size of a quarter.

As Elmer was shaving in front of the mirror one day without his shirt on, I discovered it was almost gone. The growth had lost its dark-red, shiny appearance and had shrunk to a tenth of its original size. It had turned to a normal skin tone. We knew this had happened because of his improved diet and intermittent fasting schedule.

Your Body Does it All

This chapter on therapeutic fasting emphasizes one concept: the fast, in and of itself, does nothing. The body heals itself. Fasting simply provides ideal conditions for the body to regenerate, repair, and rejuvenate itself. Out of all the fasts detailed in an earlier chapter, the absolute fast provides the most ideal conditions for the body to heal itself. By abstaining from food and taking only water, you relieve your body of digesting and eliminating a constant intake of food. Our bodies finally catch up, respond to rest, and use the energy for healing and rejuvenation.

Fasting provides the ideal conditions for the body to rejuvenate itself as the toxic buildup decreases day by day. Rest alone—even without fasting—will increase the elimination, although not nearly to the same extent. Even reducing food intake increases the excretory action. Dieters remember how many water pounds they lost during the first few days just by eliminating salty foods and sharply reducing their food intake.

To get an idea of the amount of toxin residue their bodies release during a fast, I urge fasters to take a urine specimen upon arising each day. Put it in a small, transparent jar or bottle and let it settle. Place it where the light can reflect through it. Use different containers every day to make comparisons. In a few days, you can usually observe tiny crystals forming in the urine. Notice the foreign matter that settles at the bottom of the jar. Your body does a tremendous cleansing job at the cellular level.

Undertaking a fast is the best way to allow the body to withdraw completely from alcohol, nicotine, caffeine, drugs, and toxic food. Our bodies become accustomed to certain ingested stimulants, and when we remove those stimulants—whether they be drugs or toxic foods—the body often responds with aches and pains. That's a good sign that the body is releasing toxins. This also explains the common complaint of developing a headache when a person misses his usual morning cup of coffee. The body has begun to eliminate the poisonous caffeine.

God created our bodies to heal themselves of all kinds of diseases—including the common cold. When nerve energy runs low and the bodily tissues become saturated with self-generated and self-ingested waste, the body makes a valiant attempt to eliminate the buildup. This valiant attempt is known as the common cold. The mucosal membranes throughout the system are the final avenues of elimination, and the respiratory system is affected the most.

Ideally, the cure for the common cold allows the body to self-cleanse through a short period of therapeutic fasting. Think of the money saved by avoiding doctor and drug bills! Once a person turns to healthful living practices with periodic fasting, yearly bouts with the flu, common colds, and sick days from work will be reduced or eliminated altogether. This is God's guarantee for following His natural laws of health.

Our bodies have more common sense than our educated minds! If we could but listen to our bodies when we're not well, they would scream at us, "Stop eating!" That's very wise advice. Four hundred years before Christ, Hippocrates wrote, "The more you nourish a diseased body, the worse you make it." Edward Hooker Dewey, a twentieth-century doctor, agreed. "Take away food from a sick man's stomach, and you have begun, not to starve the sick man, but the disease," he said.

As a natural, God-given instinct, our bodies don't want food when we're ill. Why? Eating actually slows the healing process. Sometimes people immediately vomit food because their bodies refuse to digest it. I remember tasting a bowl of cream of chicken soup. As soon as the first spoonful reached my stomach, the soup burst out of my mouth as if it had been shot from a gun. My body rejected the soup so quickly that I never took a second spoonful. Although the soup had spoiled in the can, I never became sick from it. Had I not vomited it immediately, I certainly would have had a bout with food poisoning.

Fasting for Weight Loss

The therapeutic fast is also the quickest and safest way to lose unwanted pounds *initially*. I emphasize initially because the weight loss is the greatest the first several days. Then it usually drops to such a disappointingly slow rate of loss that the individual would be better off eating sensibly and exercising.

In a documented case, Marie Davenport Vickers of Los Angeles, California, went on a forty-four day absolute fast. She reported that during her first three weeks, she lost twenty-two pounds. For the next three weeks, she lost only an additional two and a half pounds.[3] The human body can accomplish some amazing feats of energy conservation during fasting. This example qualifies as a record!

People often misunderstand the role of fasting in a weight-loss program. In prolonged fasting, the body's metabolism slows down. The longer the fast, the more energy conservative the human system becomes. When we stop taking in food or liquid nourishment, our bodies automatically register: "Uh-oh, famine time. Slow down." That's one reason some people can go very long without eating. The body conserves magnificently while fasting.

For weight loss, an initial few days on a fast will quickly and safety achieve the most dramatic weight loss. Dieters rejoice to see the scale go down two or three pounds a day as their bodies rapidly eliminate the salt and water. It's also a great way to get a head start on your weight-loss program. Fasting provides such a momentous weight loss at the beginning that you feel encouraged to go it on your own after the fast. These are the blessings of fasting for weight loss.

But curses also accompany fasting for weight loss. I warn you against using fasting repeatedly for weight control. The longer we deprive our bodies of nourishment, the less effective fasting becomes as a weight-loss measure. The body accustoms itself to functioning on less food by raising its starvation defenses. This makes it harder than ever to lose weight. After the fast, the body remains in this slow-metabolism, energy-conservation mode. Unless a person steps up his exercise program and cuts the calories to under 1,000 a day, this conservative metabolism will sabotage further weight loss or even halt post-fasting weight maintenance.

Eliminating Chemicals and Medicine

Dr. Paul Bragg, a life extension specialist, described his own twenty-one day, water-only fast in his book, *The Miracle of Fasting.*[4] On the tenth day, he experienced sharp pains in his bladder. When he urinated, it felt like boiling water passing through. He subsequently had his urine examined for chemicals. The examiner found traces of DDT and other deadly pesticide residue. This was in the days when the U.S. government allowed the use of DDT for spraying vegetables and fruits. DDT is now outlawed, but other deadly pesticides and herbicides are still used.

The body holds these chemicals within its tissues. Chemicals include not only the herbicides and pesticides pumped into our toxic food supply, but also all the over-the-counter drugs and prescription medicines you have ever taken.

The drugs from the pharmaceutical world are unnatural, anti-vital poisons that lower your nerve energy and set the stage for acute and chronic disease. They should be released from the body. Incidentally, there is no medical way to release chemicals from the body. They stay trapped in the body for years. With the aid of the fast, their release can be achieved. The medical world does not recognize that drugs are that toxic, nor does it validate that the body will eliminate these drugs while fasting. The hopes of becoming drug-free with standard medical treatment are nil.

Paul Bragg believes that he restored his health from tuberculosis through systematic fasting. He became such a believer in fasting that he fasted once a week and went on longer ten-day fasts four times a year. After five years of systematic fasting, Bragg was enjoying a quiet ride in a canoe when he suddenly doubled up with stomach cramps and hurriedly paddled to shore. His bowels evacuated and ended with a heavy, cool sensation in the rectum. A chemist examined his stool and discovered Bragg had passed a third of a cup of quicksilver (mercury) from the calomel medicine his mother had given him for whooping cough during his childhood.[5]

As you know by now, the longer the fast, the more the body expels. One fast alone will not detoxify everything that your body has stored for many years—unless your fast is the completed fast mentioned in an earlier chapter. Several short fasts may produce the most effective results for you.

Persevere during Your Fast

Occasionally, some people resist the idea of fasting for health because they assume their condition is too complicated or too severe. Once an individual educates himself in fasting, such instances tend to be the exception. As statistics prove, the overwhelming percentage of persons helped with therapeutic fasting far exceeds any other kind of care available. Coupled with faith in God, through prayer and fasting we have the most powerful source of healing for our physical bodies. We must educate ourselves and then persevere.

Discomfort sometimes occurs during a fast. When people complain of pain while fasting in a fasting institute, we encourage them with the following statements.

"Be glad! You're getting rid of poisons!" "Something good is happening." "Relax! Your body is doing some deep cleaning."

When people go on fasts to receive healing, we urge them, "Don't let your faith in God waver when the discomforting symptoms prevail. You must persevere. Your body is in pain, but this pain is not the pain of disease. This is the pain of healing. This pain is your friend. Your body is healing itself as a result of this fast. As your body breaks down and eliminates the toxins, you may not feel so great."

Of course, not everyone experiences pain and discomfort. These unpleasant moments are usually short-lived. This is a small price to pay to avoid the surgeon's knife, dangerous drugs, and costly hospital bills.

Amazing Results with Fasting

Hippocrates, the father of medicine, lived four hundred years before Christ. This wise doctor often prescribed fasting to combat illness. We should consider one of his many timely quotes: "Everyone has a doctor within him. We just have to help this doctor in his work." Practicing what he preached, Hippocrates lived to the ripe old age of ninety.

Over the years, I've collected information on fasting experiences and experiments. These records of rejuvenation and healing through fasting show the miracle-working power of the body to cleanse and heal itself. God didn't leave out any important detail in His wonderful masterpiece.

According to their figures, the staff at the McEachen Sanatorium in Escondido, California, supervised the fasting of 715 people between August 1952 and March 1958. The only limitation in the efficiency of treatment was that many patients did not have time to fast long enough or often enough to obtain maximum benefit. Fasting these 715 people yielded the following results:

- 294 cases showed great improvement or complete recovery
- 360 experienced moderate benefit
- 61 reported no improvement

In other words, an overwhelming 88.4 percent improved or totally recovered. If only modern-day medical care could present such statistics to the American people![6]

Dr. William L. Esser, one of the world's leading natural hygienic practitioners, has a retreat in West Palm Beach, Florida. He reported fasting 156 people who collectively complained of symptoms from thirty-one medically diagnosed diseases, including ulcers, tumors, tuberculosis, sinusitis, pyorrhea, Parkinson's disease, heart disease, cancer, insomnia, gallstones, epilepsy, colitis, hay fever, bronchitis, asthma, and arthritis. The shortest fast among these 156 patients lasted five days, and the longest lasted fifty-five.

In spite of only 20 percent of the patients remaining in his sanatorium to fast as long as Dr. Esser recommended, their results were, nevertheless, totally astounding when compared with the standard medical treatment:

- 113 completely recovered
- 31 partially recovered
- 12 were not helped

Ninety-two percent improved or totally recovered! Do you wonder why more people don't understand the benefits of fasting? Many medical doctors and pharmacists would have to take down their shingle if this secret gets out.

Psychiatrist Dr. Allan Cott used fasting as a treatment for schizophrenics and reported his results in *Applied Nutrition in Clinical Practice.*[7] Dr. Cott placed twenty-eight patients on an absolute fast at the Gracie Square Hospital in New York. All patients had been diagnosed as schizophrenic for at least five years and had not responded to standard treatment. Dr. Cott reported remarkable success in 60 percent of the cases.

The author who reported on this experiment and who also took a cautious view of fasting admitted that great promise lies in fasting the mentally ill:

> At present…it seems that fasting is of the most practical use in cases of schizophrenia, where other treatments have not worked. It is always possible, of course, that further work will show that if fasting is given as the primary treatment rather than the treatment of last resort, it will be found to be extremely useful.[8]

Dr. Shelton's Health School, the world's most famous natural hygiene institution ever run, saw 40,000 patients from 1928 to 1981. In 1964, Dr. Shelton published the most famous book on the therapeutic fast ever sold: *Fasting Can Save Your Life.* Shelton, however, wrote from the vantage point of fasting as a pure science. *Fasting Can Save Your Life* is an easily read, easily understood book full of remarkable case histories on the value of therapeutic fasting. I highly recommend it for your library.

Dr. Shelton's book claims that the treatment of virtually every acute or chronic disease responds with astounding success to properly supervised fasting. Just some of the diseases discussed in detail are the common cold, multiple sclerosis, asthma, arthritis, ulcers, migraines, hay fever, cardiovascular disease, obesity, colitis, psoriasis, eczema, tumors, gallstones, and more. This book gives great encouragement that the therapeutic fast can help your body recover without drugs.

Elmer's Bout with the Amoebas

When Elmer and I lived in the Canal Zone, Elmer experienced an unusual turn of events during a five-day fast. For seven years he had suffered from amoebas that had settled in his intestinal tract. He had acquired them during our many years of missionary work in less-than-sanitary conditions in foreign countries. Every four or five days for nearly seven years, he went through a cycle of diarrhea. He suffered with the same symptoms that hit many people when they travel. This always left him weak and nearly lifeless.

Elmer had subjected himself to many tests at the Stanford Medical Center in Palo Alto, California, as well as the Gorgas Hospital in the Canal Zone, where the doctors are experts with tropical diseases. He had been to many other doctors and clinics and had tried all their suggestions. He was even given morphine at one time to paralyze his bowels. Nothing worked. The doctors gave him the classic response: "You'll just have to learn to live with it."

On the fourth night of an absolute fast, taken for spiritual reasons, Elmer was delivered from his miserable bout with the amoebas. His body perspired so profusely that we had to change the bed covers. His severe cramps rushed him to the bathroom. We did not know much about fasting and wondered why, after not eating for four days, he had to have a bowel movement. After the bowels evacuated, Elmer immediately felt better. Since that day, more than fifteen years ago, he has never had another bout with amoebas.

The doctors who examined Elmer at Stanford University told us that the amoebas laid eggs that hatched every three to four days. Each time this occurred, his body tried to expel the irritating parasites, resulting in diarrhea.

Hearing the doctors' explanations, we concluded that the fast had starved the amoebas. With nothing to feed on and with the excretory organs accelerating their activity during the fast, the amoebas could no longer live in his body. Elmer's body—more fully detoxified and more charged with healing nerve energy—was no longer a hospitable environment for disease-promoting organisms. He had not only fasted himself but the amoebas as well!

Regain Your Health—and Keep It!

Therapeutic fasting is most beneficial to those who are sick and want to get well without drugs and doctors. Therapeutic fasting, however, should also be viewed as a modern form of disease prevention and health maintenance.

For the sick person, fasting should become the favored means to restore health. For the healthy person, fasting should become the favored form of health insurance.

Undertaking a fast when you're seriously ill often brings amazing results. When a person turns to fasting in the earlier stages of illness, the results come easier. More wisdom lies in prevention and maintenance than in removing a disease.

The novice may find it hard to believe that fasting could be of such great benefit to those suffering from a wide variety of diseases. From what we have learned, however, it should not be surprising at all. According to the theory of natural hygiene, toxemia causes all disease. We must remove that one cause and provide the ideal conditions for health. Experience shows us that the fast is the most powerful of those ideal conditions for health restoration.

Someone who does not understand these basic laws of physiology may find it hard to believe that one simple, inexpensive, short-lived, therapeutic technique could work virtual miracles in the lives of nearly every sick person fighting for his life today! My life-or-death adventure gave me irrefutable personal experience. I have also seen documented reports where people have been healed or greatly helped by fasting in such sicknesses as colitis, acne, arthritis, gout, headaches, liver and kidney troubles, ulcerated teeth, and measles.

We need to understand that these are not localized diseases caused by some attacking germ or virus. These local manifestations reflect a general condition throughout the body caused by one factor—toxemia. Understanding this, we can see that the location of the symptom makes no difference. By removing the cause—which is toxemia throughout the system—and by providing the conditions for health—which are fasting and healthful living practices—the symptoms disappear. Health is restored.

Many of Dr. Shelton's 40,000 patients whom he fasted had been given up as hopeless by their own doctors. In spite of this fact, an amazingly high percentage of these "incurables" either greatly improved or fully restored their health at Dr. Shelton's Health School. As reported in *Therapeutic Fasting,* "The percentage of recoveries has been amazingly high—exceeding that resulting from the use of any other therapeutic measure."[9]

We cannot live as long as the early generations of mankind, partially because of our polluted, stress-filled, modern lifestyles; but we can revise our living habits. We can improve the quality of our day-to-day living and ultimately extend our lives, enjoying increasing levels of health by using the fast as one of our revised living habits.

Life does not have to be a gamble, lived only by chance. God has given us some of the responsibility for our own life span. We are not living victoriously until we learn and practice God's laws instead of breaking them. We must take control of the conditions that threaten to destroy us and reverse them.

To live in ignorance is to live in slavery. But Scripture teaches, *"The law of the wise is a fountain of life, to turn one away from the snares of death"* (Proverbs 13:14). Wisdom comes through knowledge, and knowledge comes from seeking the truth. The Bible promises, *"Seek, and you will find"* (Matthew 7:7).

Once we understand and obey God's natural health laws, we can truly experience the abundant life that Jesus Christ promises. (See John 10:10.) The Bible also says that if you fast correctly, *"Then your light shall break forth like the morning, your healing shall spring forth speedily, and your righteousness shall go before you"* (Isaiah 58:8). Through fasting and prayer we can regain our health—and keep it!

Eight

Fasting for a Longer Life

The last chapter pointed out that the therapeutic fast brings about great physical healing. As the body cleanses its fluids and tissues and eliminates toxins, we experience a new vitality. A more youthful appearance is a natural fringe benefit of fasting. Being rejuvenated by fasting contrasts with futile attempts at drinking from the fountain of youth.

Early in the fifteenth century, Juan Ponce de Leon sought the fountain of youth in the land he discovered called Bimini, which he later named Florida. Ever since that time, men and women have spent fortunes seeking a cure for aging.

In 1954, the late Dr. Ana Aslan, a Nobel Prize winner for her work and director of the Institute of Geriatrics in Bucharest, Romania, reported in the *Journal of Romanian Academy of Science* her findings of an antiaging vitamin compound. Nikita Khrushchev, John F. Kennedy, the Gabors, and thousands of others have flown to Romania for her famous antiaging treatments.

On February 10, 1986, Dr. Christian Barnard and biologists at the Schaefer Institute in Switzerland began to market a new product in five hundred American department stores. They called it Glycel and hailed it as an antiaging cream that encourages the skin to regenerate. Dermatologists were skeptical, and only time could determine its success. According to a news release in *USA Today,* Glycel's key ingredients are a group of chemicals called GSL, short for glycosphingolipids, found in youthful skin but less abundant in older people. In recent years, dermatologists have been promoting the virtues of a substance called Retin-A, purported to give the skin a youthful glow and reduce tiny wrinkles in the skin.

Tecopa Hot Springs, a small desert town near Death Valley, California, is one of many health spas that boasts of its natural, hot, healing, mineral waters. Each year, thousands soak in its supposed healing and rejuvenating waters. There have been and still are magic potions, as well as healing waters and countless other so-called rejuvenating methods, to which the masses flock in their vain attempts to restore their health and regain their youth. Unfortunately, their success is usually minimal, if they have any at all.

Exercise

Many people find the next best thing to the fountain of youth is a regular program of vigorous exercise. Scientific studies show that exercise is, without a doubt, a powerfully rejuvenating lifestyle habit. The exercise industry promotes itself with well-founded claims of longevity and has boomed into a multi-billion dollar business in America. Health clubs are thriving, packed with classes on stretching and toning, rebounding, gymnastics and swimnastics, aerobic dance with weights, and sophisticated supplemental machines to help build a body to look like Mr. Universe or Miss America.

Elmer and I witnessed this exercise boom in our own community. Not long ago, we lived in a resort area right on the beach. Whenever I left for my daily six-mile walk, whether I got up before sunrise or waited until dusk, the walkers, joggers, skaters, and cyclers were already out in full force.

In the late 1960s, when Elmer and I lived in Costa Rica, passersby ridiculed and jeered Elmer for his jogging because they couldn't understand why a person would run just for the sake of running. He finally decided to take our Doberman pinscher with him. No one made fun of him. They thought it was perfectly fine to exercise his dog. Times have changed, however. Today, visitors to the beautiful Central American country of Costa Rica might see entire streets blocked off so runners can exercise freely. Even there they've taken up this exercise craze.

The idea of recapturing health, vitality, and youthfulness is, admittedly, attractive. Throughout the ages, men and women have even harbored the secret, albeit unrealistic, desire for life everlasting here on earth. Instances of historical searches for the fountain of youth abound, as do their present-day counterparts. Only a few of these pursuits are valid, however. All of them, without exception, are found in the healthful living practices detailed in this book.

Sin and Aging

The book of Genesis implies that God originally created our bodies to live forever. We lost this ability through disobedience in the Garden of Eden. The same day that Adam and Eve ate of the Tree of Knowledge of Good and Evil, the penalty of death took effect. Adam and Eve and their descendants were destined to die one day.

Once the first couple sinned, God didn't want Adam and Eve to eat of the Tree of Life. If this had happened, they would have been condemned to live in their physical, sinful state forever. To prevent this, God cast them out of the Garden of Eden. (See Genesis 3:22–24.)

Although God pronounced death upon the human race from that point in history, people lived in good health and to what seem to be incredible ages. Here are some amazing examples of longevity:

- Adam lived 930 years and fathered a child at the age of 130. (See Genesis 5:3–5.)
- Methuselah, who boasts the longest recorded life span of 969 years, became a father for the first time at age 187. (See Genesis 5:25, 27.)
- Noah was 500 years old when he fathered Shem. (See Genesis 5:32.)

From Adam to Noah, the life span averaged 912 years. Within eight generations of Noah, however, the average length of life diminished to around 148 years—a startling decline of 802 years. Within eight generations, the human race lost nearly 85 percent of its life expectancy.

Throughout the ages, death and dying have filled the human race with horror. (This horror is, of course, more pronounced among unbelievers.) As a result, people frantically search for the fountain of youth or some such secret to prolong life. From a theological perspective, Christians know why we will one day die. We have sinned. Disobedience eventually cuts off life for every one of us.

What is God's promise regarding the human life span? Many Christians say that the answer to this question lies in Moses' statement:

> *The days of our lives are seventy years; and if by reason of strength they are eighty years, yet their boast is only labor and sorrow; for it is soon cut off, and we fly away.* (Psalm 90:10)

Those who point to this verse as proof of our limited life spans are mistaken. These believers think that we will live only seventy years, or if we're in exceptional health, eighty. They conclude that if we survive beyond seventy, we are living on borrowed time.

I don't agree. During the time of this writing, the Israelites were living under a curse in the wilderness. (See Numbers 14:29–37.) God had shortened their lives so that the old, faithless generation would die within forty years. This made it possible for them to number their days. (See Psalms 90:12.) This reference cannot define God's allotted life span for people today. God never said, "You shall live only seventy or eighty years." Besides that, Moses himself lived to be 120. Faithful Caleb didn't even enter the promised land until he was 80.

If this verse wasn't written for modern Christians, then what is God's projection for our life span? No one can say for certain, but one thing is sure. If we didn't break God's natural laws of physical, emotional, mental, and spiritual health, we could easily live much longer and in much better condition. Violating God's laws results in enervation, toxemia, and increasing stages of disease. Youthfulness and longevity are finally lost to sickness and death.

How We Poison Ourselves

Through the buildup of toxins, we poison ourselves in small doses every day. Our autointoxication brings on disease and reduces longevity. Let's look at the two types of toxins and their sources. First, our bodies create *endogenous toxins* as a result of:

1. Metabolic waste: ongoing, toxic by-products at the cellular level
2. Spent debris from cellular activities
3. Dead cells
4. Emotional and mental distress and excess
5. Physical fatigue, distress, and excess

Second, *exogenous toxins* are man-made toxins that we ingest. Some of the sources for these toxins include:

1. Unnatural food and drink
2. Natural food denatured by cooking, refining, and preserving
3. Improper food combinations
4. Medical, pharmaceutical, and herbal drugging
5. Tobacco, alcohol, and recreational drugging
6. Environmental, commercial, and industrial pollutants
7. Impure air and water

We pollute our air, our water, and our environment. The food industrialists contaminate our foods for a longer shelf life. Toxins pervert our appetites, encouraging us to eat beyond natural hunger. Advertisers brainwash us to build our diets around synthetic and junk foods. Because of our sedentary lifestyles and refusal to exercise, we develop hypokinetic diseases. We flood our minds with killing emotions as we cope with the stresses of life. When God created the Garden of Eden, He did not intend for His children to live like this!

What Life Extensionists Say

Despite the increase in life expectancy over the centuries, experts in longevity now say that the maximum age reached by a few people has not changed. Our maximum life span, determined by our biological clock, seems to be about 115 to 120 years—providing that we cultivate healthy lifestyles.

Some researchers are challenging that. The latest theory in the field, now called life extension, holds that one day we will be able to prolong human life to 140 years. They base this on their theory that they can learn to slow down the biological rate of aging.

Other advocates of life extension don't suggest we can have more years. But they do foresee a better quality life by learning to push back the age at which the manifestations of aging and chronic diseases first appear. Pushing back the aging process means we must practice health maintenance effectively.

One expert in a televised interview predicted the possibilities for longevity enhancement:

> I can foresee aging without debilitating disease to about age 100, possibly 110, but not much more. Even if we could eliminate the chronic killers, such as cancer and heart disease, we would gain only about twelve years. If we find a way to extend life, it will, in my opinion, come through intervening in the aging process itself by slowing it down.

While the average life expectancy for men in the United States is 74 and for women is 76, many Americans today are, nevertheless, living beyond the century mark. Our country boasts about 32,000 centenarians.

Doctors still give quotes that smack of the fountain of youth. Dr. Friedenburg, a noted physician from New York, optimistically stated, "With a perfectly balanced endocrine system, man would live forever."[1] Another doctor has reflected, "The human frame as a machine is perfect. It contains within itself no marks by which we can possibly predict its decay. It was apparently intended to go on forever."[2]

Theories of Aging

Why do people gradually grow old, lose their muscle tone, and become increasing susceptible to life-threatening disease? The current popular theories on what causes the human body to age fall into the two following broad categories:

The *damage theory of aging* describes the random damage from outside agents as a by-product of our own metabolism. Theoretically, this position says that if we could eliminate these random damages or repair them perfectly, it would prolong the length and quality of life.

One example of such damage is cross-linking. We grow stiff with age, much like a rubber band that no longer stretches. A cross-linking agent (in the form of a chemical) takes hold of two separate molecules or two parts of the same molecule and binds them together. These agents are churned out as by-products of normal metabolism. They are also the result of molecules that enter the body in the form of exogenous toxins, such as unnatural food and drink, recreational and medicinal drugs, and pollution.

Another example of damage is a free radical. The theory says that extra electrons from unstable molecules will aggressively seek other molecules on which to attach themselves. Free radicals have been likened to great white sharks in the biochemical sea. Researchers have implicated these destructive free radicals in cancer, arteriosclerosis, hypertension, Alzheimer's disease, and AIDS.

The *program theory* explains aging as genetically planned obsolescence. These researchers believe that we have the equivalent of pre-programmed aging clocks inside our bodies. Let's look at three time-programmed theories:

The *cellular clock theory* says that each cell in the body has a genetic clock that ticks away, so to speak, until it reaches its limit. Researchers at the University of Florida have substantiated this theory. Since the 1960s, they have observed that cells will not divide to renew themselves more than fifty times. The cellular clock theory seeks ways to increase the number of cellular divisions possible in the life of each cell.

The *neuroendocrine theory* investigates the possibility of a sudden-death hormone that the pituitary gland releases or that results from a slowly developing hormonal imbalance. Advocates of this theory are intrigued that the endocrine glands (such as thyroid, pancreas, pituitary, and testes) tend to shrink with age and exhibit age-related declines in the secretion of hormones. For example, women have a sharp drop in estrogen secretion during menopause. These hormonal changes may be programmed in the brain. The neuroendocrine theory purports that we have a clock in the brain and another in each cell that controls the aging process, and these theorists are seeking new ways to reprogram these clocks.

The *immune system theory* notes that, as we age, the immune system functions less efficiently and fails to protect us from autointoxication and from offending bacteria and viruses. This theory seeks to extend life by finding ways to strengthen the immune system.

Life Extension and the Blood

A few researchers are attempting to explain aging by combining the foregoing theories. I find it interesting that most of these theories depend upon the circulation of the blood. While I am no expert in the aging research, I know the Bible declares, *"The life of the flesh is in the blood"* (Leviticus 17:11). Although this information was available in the Bible for thousands of years, William Harvey didn't discover that the blood circulates through arteries and veins until 1618.

The cardiocirculatory system, a vast transportation system throughout the body, has many functions. Its primary function, however, is to carry gases and minute particles through nearly 100,000 miles of tubing to all parts of the body: carrying nourishment to the cells and waste products away from the cells so that they may live, excrete, repair, multiply, and thrive.

The ancient Greeks believed and taught in their medical schools that the arteries were simple air tubes. They concluded this upon always finding the arteries empty when they examined the human corpse. Arteries were thus named "artere," meaning the "air." The Grecian teachings went undisputed as the empirical truth throughout the ages until Dr. Harvey announced his findings.

Medical doctors scoffed at Harvey's discovery that the blood circulated throughout the arterial and venal systems. Historian Wilder Hume wrote, "No physician in Europe who had reached the age of forty, ever to the end of his life, adopted Harvey's doctrine of the circulation of the blood."[3] Dr. William H. Hay reported that Harvey's peers ridiculed him at first; but when they were unable to disprove his statement, they were filled with rage. They organized a system of persecution against him until they broke his heart.[4] Although circulation of the blood is an undisputed scientific fact today, the idea that the purity of the bloodstream may hold the key to youthfulness and longevity is seldom a consideration.

If it's true that our bodies could exist forever or that human life could be greatly extended beyond the average seventy-five years of age, then why do we age and eventually die? The renowned scientist Mitchnikoff stated, "Deterioration of bodily structure and old age are due to poisonous substances in the blood."[5] Dr. James

Empringham, who lived at the turn of the twentieth century, believed that all creatures automatically poison themselves. He taught that toxic products in the blood produced the senile changes we call old age.

If the hygienists' toxemia theory of disease is correct, as Mitchnikoff and Empringham and I concur, then the very same blood that gives us life can also carry disease. Disease and premature death come only because our wrong living habits have polluted the bloodstream beyond its toleration point. Our metabolic waste and ingested toxins accumulate in the blood. As a result, we irritate, inflame, and poison our delicate cells. The continual overload can only lead to degenerative disease, premature aging, and death.

Our bodies are wonderfully designed. Billions and billions of red corpuscles flow through the bloodstream. When our nerve energy is sapped and toxemia sets in, disease soon follows. We often experience stagnated circulation and weak blood. How can we improve blood quality and accelerate our circulation? These functions are supplied within the body and by the body. Only the body can make blood and keep it pure. Even the wisest chemist cannot make a drop.

Likewise, only the body can recharge its nerve energy so that it has the power to purify the bodily fluids and tissues. Self-cure, therefore, is also the only cure possible. Any change of living habits that allows conditions for rest and fasting, followed by right eating, exercise, sunbathing, emotional balance, spiritual well-being, and all the other essentials of health will contribute to the reparative process.

David wrote in praise of God and His fabulous handiwork when he sang,

> *You made all the delicate, inner parts of my body, and knit them together in my mother's womb. Thank you for making me so wonderfully complex! It is amazing to think about. Your workmanship is marvelous—and how well I know it.*
> (Psalm 139:13–14 TLB)

Does the secret to long life lie in keeping the blood and bodily fluids pure and free of toxic material? French physician and biologist Alexis Carrel of the Rockefeller Institute discovered the method of transplantation of organs. From his studies, he formally declared,

> The cell is immortal. It is merely the fluid in which it floats that degenerates. Renew this fluid at proper intervals, and give the cell nourishment upon which to feed, and so far as we know, the pulsation of life may go on forever.[6]

Dr. Carrel experimented with keeping tissues and organs, separate from the body yet alive, under various laboratory conditions. He confirmed his declaration on the immortality of the cell through an experiment in which he kept a chicken heart alive for twenty-eight years. Since the life span of a chicken is only eight to ten years, Dr. Carrel's story is quite remarkable.

Dr. Carrel pointed out the reason for his chicken heart's longevity. As long as the nutrients fed to the heart were pure and the constantly produced metabolic wastes of elimination were washed away so that the cells were never clogged, then the heart could live in excellent condition. Furthermore, he concluded that the heart would die only if the waste accumulated to toxic levels. The heart did die, but only because Dr. Carrel decided to end his long-term nurturing of the chicken heart and turn his attention elsewhere.

Dr. Carrel's findings suggest that old age comes about because of minute quantities of poisonous substances in the blood. The body renews and replenishes the blood continually. Given the ideal conditions for health, would Dr. Carrel's chicken heart have lived forever?

Another Longevity Experiment

The son of Julian Huxley isolated a worm whose normal life span is three months long. He alternately fed it restricted amounts of foods followed by periods of fasting. It was still alive and vigorous after nineteen generations of its relatives had been born, lived their normal life spans, and died! Dr. Huxley concluded that heavy eating clogs the life channels and hastens death, but fasting allows the body to rejuvenate by self-purification.[7]

Extrapolate the results of Huxley's experiment and apply them to the human race. If a man who might ordinarily die at fifty could likewise extend his life by nineteen times, he would live 950 years. This was the age to which Noah lived. (See Genesis 9:29.) Perhaps those remarkable ages to which people lived in the early days of the Bible were not so hyperbolic after all!

Let's examine another case. Doctors Carlson and Knude of the Department of Physiology at the University of Chicago placed a forty-year-old man on a fourteen-day fast. At the end of the fast, they examined his tissues and declared that they were of the same physiological condition as those of a seventeen-year-old youth.

Dr. Knude stated, "It is evident that where the initial weight was reduced by 45 percent, and subsequently restored by normal diet, approximately one-half of the restored body is made up of new protoplasm. In this, there is rejuvenescence."[8]

Dr. Herbert M. Shelton, author of *Fasting Can Save Your Life,* wholeheartedly agrees. Here's what he wrote:

> Fasting can bring about a virtual "rebirth," a revitalization of the organism. As the fast progresses, all of the cells of the body undergo refinement, and there is a removal from the protoplasm of the cells of stored, foreign substances so that cells become more youthful and function more efficiently.
>
> Anyone experienced with fasting has seen great numbers of instances of physical rejuvenation achieved by means of the fast. The mental improvements commonly match the physical improvements. Occasional restoration of hearing in ears that have been deaf for years, improved vision, discarding glasses that have been worn for years, increased acuity of the senses of taste and smell, restoration of ability to sense delicate flavors, recovery of the sense of feeling in instances of sensory paralysis, stepped-up vigor, increased mental powers, loss of weight, greatly increased functional vigor, with better digestion and better bowel action, clear and sparkling eyes, clearing of the complexion with a restoration of youthful bloom, the disappearance of some of the finer lines of the face, reduced blood pressure, better heart action, reduction of enlarged prostate, sexual rejuvenation—these and many other evidences of rejuvenation are seen by everyone who has a wide experience with fasting.[9]

The restorative, rejuvenating effects of a fast commonly affect the five senses of the faster. Sight, smell, hearing, taste, and touch all show marked sensitivity. This, of course, is a delight to the post-faster, as all senses are heightened and all enjoyment increased.

The sense of smell improves so much that fasters tell me they find themselves nauseated by foul odors they scarcely noticed before. One lady wrote me that her friend decided to go on a short fast. The friend hadn't been able to smell anything for years. After only four days, she was able to smell again. But this process works in reverse, too. Once the friend returned to her former poor eating habits, her sense of smell was again dulled; eventually she lost it completely.

Allowing the body to houseclean during a fast could be promoted as the closest thing to a health panacea on the market. Let me describe some of the physical changes that a fast can cause in a diseased body.

The complexion often clears beautifully with a fast, and difficult acne problems are often lessened or eliminated. Lines and wrinkles soften or disappear; blotches, discolorations, and pimples become less apparent or disappear. The general tone of the skin becomes more youthful with better color and texture. The whites of the eyes become so white that they sparkle. The eyes take on such a brightness and clear quality that people often remark how alive you look. People just look younger after fasting.

Mahatma Gandhi was known for his many fasts. On May 18, 1933, physicians examined him on the tenth day of one of his fasts. His doctor marveled that despite Gandhi's sixty-four years of age, he was as healthy as a man of forty.

The scientific community is now accepting physical regeneration as a scientific fact. The rejuvenating effects of a wholesome, conservative diet and a program of alternate fasting turn on the fountain of youth within our own bodies.

Unfortunately, many of us still eat the way the American homesteaders did when they worked hard from dawn to dusk and needed hearty meals to tackle intense physical activity. While the level of our physical activity no longer warrants heavy food intake, we eat like the pioneers. This invites enervation and toxemia and leads us into the stages of disease.

Fasting is God's way of providing the ideal conditions that allow the body to purify its blood, cells, tissues, and organs. By relieving the body of the processes of ingesting, chewing, swallowing, digesting, metabolizing, and eliminating nutrients, the blood can do a thorough job of cleaning itself.

By withholding food from the body and resting at the same time, we restore the nerve energy that the body needs in order to eliminate the toxic overload at the cellular level. This is the true process of self-purification. It's also the only way—God's way—to achieve longevity and to drink at the fountain of youth.

Nine

Eating to Live or Living to Eat?

What's uppermost in the minds of most Americans? If you immediately thought of sex, you missed it. When interviewed in a popular magazine, actor Jack Lemmon pointed out that we see sex flaunted in magazines, newspapers, on television, radio, and billboards. But the number one thing on the minds of Americans is not sex. It's food.

We think about food constantly. We build our social lives around eating. Many business people have discovered that sales pitches work wonders when customers have food placed in front of them. We hardly finish one meal before we plan the next. We seldom meet friends just to be together; we usually plan our gatherings around food. Almost without exception, we socialize around a meal. Or we add a refreshment, a snack, or "a bite to eat" to the social agenda. If it's not food that makes the centerpiece of our relationships, it's a beverage. We issue the standard invitations: "Let's meet for coffee," or "Let's have a drink."

A punster of the nineteenth century quipped, "Armies travel on their bellies." So do we. One food expert commented that the deal between people and the government is an economic one, and food supply stands at the top of the list.

When Our Bellies Become Our Gods

Controlling our sex lives is easier than limiting our intake of food. Uncontrolled eating sneaks into our lives. We nibble. We decide to have our coffee black (or with artificial sweetener). Without thinking, we treat ourselves to a doughnut or slice of cake to go along with our coffee. The urge to eat out of habit—not hunger—slips into our minds in the most subtle ways.

Eating is, admittedly, enjoyable; the act of eating satisfies more needs than simple hunger. For example, Mom fed us when we cried. She rewarded us with a piece of candy when we were good. When we received an honor, she baked a cake. In later years, we learned to mother ourselves by indulging in our favorite meal whenever we felt deserving.

Can you imagine any organization giving out awards without planning a banquet? Can you imagine a church that doesn't have a social gathering centered on food—and lots of it? How many church groups, such as the missionary society, meet regularly and don't serve refreshments?

When our seams feel tight and our belts need to be loosened, we know we need to do something about our excess weight. All too often, however, we excuse ourselves. As we enjoy those extra calories, we jokingly remark to anyone who happens to notice, "I'll have to run around the block a couple of times to make up for this." (Actually, running a mile burns only ninety calories. We would have to jog up to ten miles for some of the sweet desserts we consume!)

Our obsession with food is bad enough from a nutritional perspective. But for Christians, overindulgence is more than added calories, flabby stomachs, and bulging thighs. It is sin—a subtle sin, but still sin. Our lack of self-control damages God's holy temples—our bodies. (See 1 Corinthians 3:16–17; 6:19–20; 10:31.)

If we're honest, most of us will admit that food is a controlling force in our lives—a little god that wields awful power. We no longer eat to live, but we truly live to eat. If we doubt that, we only have to step back and view our world. Over half the people in America today are obese or near obese.[1] According to the U.S. Department of Public Health, over eighty million Americans are more than 20 percent overweight; as many as 75 percent of all adult Americans may be at least ten pounds overweight.[2]

Barry Tarshis, author of *The Average American,* estimates the number of obese Americans ranges somewhere between 25 to 40 percent of the population, with more women than men and more lower than higher income individuals fitting into that category.[3] Results from a 1985 survey conducted by *Better Homes and Gardens* estimates that 65.5 percent of all Americans started a diet that year. The same survey said that 70 percent of us think we have at least five pounds to lose.

Not only have we let our bellies become our gods, but we're also killing ourselves with "the good life." Just because some people aren't overweight doesn't mean they are not guilty of overindulgence. A person doesn't have to be obese in order to be toxic. People who are normal weight or even underweight are sometimes just as susceptible to enervation and toxemia as overweight individuals.

Americans believe that they must eat three square meals a day. For many, those three meals have been converted to one meal a day, beginning in the morning and ending just before going to bed. We force our digestive machines to churn, constantly overworking and overwhelming them into early exhaustion. We've learned that exhaustion leads to enervation and toxemia, which set the stage for the descent into disease.

In his book *Shape Up,* Dr. Quein Hyder warns us of the health hazards of obesity:

> Obesity is by far the most common single sign of physical unfitness in America. It is the natural result of the combination of gluttony and physical inactivity and is most common in middle life. It is a grim predictor of serious illness to come. Although being overweight per se is not potentially fatal, it is associated with a variety of medical conditions which do shorten life. For example, it is almost always a common denominator in most heart diseases, high blood pressure, arteriosclerosis, diabetes, gall bladder disease, and shortness of breath. Obesity may actually result from certain disorders of metabolism, the endocrine glands, or the central nervous system; but these are all very rare.[4]

Despite statistics that reveal Americans are living longer, don't be fooled! Government statistics average all births and deaths. A significant decrease in infant mortality has lengthened the expected life span. But people are not living any longer today than they did two hundred years ago.

Ministers of the Gospel, lay workers, and believers from all walks of life are aging prematurely, suffering disease needlessly, and dying an early death. We often console ourselves and say, "God took him." But it was not necessarily God who took our loved ones. These people helped to plant the seeds of toxemia that led to fatal tissue degeneration. Whether they realized it or not, their lifestyle became responsible for an untimely death.

The Bible also says, *"My people are destroyed for lack of knowledge"* (Hosea 4:6). After reading this book, you'll no longer lack the knowledge for a long, healthy, and satisfying life. Even with this knowledge, many will find it difficult to change. Addiction does not die easily. Think about the cigarette smokers who know that their habit is the number one cause of lung cancer, yet they continue to puff away. Changing our eating habits may be equally challenging. But once we change, we will add years to our lives.

When we continue our poor eating styles, we suffer from a host of food-induced sicknesses. Obesity itself, developed from a steady diet of too much food and a poor quality of food, aggravates and precipitates virtually every other known disease. Even if a person does not become obese, eating steadily from the standard American diet inevitably brings disease.

Until we study the health hazards of the standard American diet, we will remain in ignorance. Stop denying that your wrong eating habits are causing your illness, and enjoy the blessings of God's natural foods.

Take responsibility for your own physical well-being by becoming a living example of health in the Lord.

Overindulgence is one of the most serious sins of modern Americans, whether it takes place in the form of trying to "keep up with the Joneses" or by physically trying to satisfy every carnal craving. "Lust of the eyes" and "lust of the flesh" (see 1 John 2:16)—Americans have it all—and shamefully so. Our lifestyles make Paul's words relevant for today:

> *Their future is eternal loss, for their god is their appetite: they are proud of what they should be ashamed of; and all they think about is this life here on earth.* (Philippians 3:19 TLB)

On the other hand, Jesus taught us to follow Him, rather than our own carnal desires:

> *Do not worry about your life, what you will eat or what you will drink; nor about your body, what you will put on. Is not life more than food and the body more than clothing?* (Matthew 6:25)

Our Original Downfall

Remember mankind's first sin? Satan enticed Adam and Eve to eat the forbidden fruit:

> *And the serpent said to the woman, "You will not surely die. For God knows that in the day you eat of it your eyes will be opened, and you will be like God, knowing good and evil."*
> (Genesis 3:4–5)

Satan tempted them with food! From the beginning, Satan began to attack our most vulnerable area.

> *So when the woman saw that the tree was good for food, that it was pleasant to the eyes, and a tree desirable to make one wise, she took of its fruit and ate. She also gave to her husband with her, and he ate.* (Genesis 3:6)

Look at the steps to temptation. They are no different from the way the power of food works today:

1. The food looked delicious.
2. Satan enticed Adam and Eve so that they desired the food beyond their better judgment.
3. Once they rationalized their action, they indulged in the forbidden food and suffered deadly consequences.

Having succeeded in the Garden of Eden, Satan has used food throughout the history of God's people to bring them to ruin and destruction. The Bible records several examples of fleshly cravings and the disastrous results of not restraining them.

When Esau arrived home exhausted from a hunting trip, he looked at the pot of stew his brother Jacob was cooking and asked for some. Knowing how much his brother liked to eat, Jacob persuaded Esau to trade his birthright for a bowl of stew. He responded to Jacob with a vow to sell his most precious earthly treasure, his inheritance rights as the eldest son. In those days, the firstborn son received a double inheritance and the richest blessings. (See Genesis 25:29–34.)

The record of the Jewish nation wandering in the wilderness is also a tale about being ruined by the lust for food. The people yearned to return to Egypt, where they had a diet rich in meats, onions, leeks, and garlic.

When God rained down quail to satisfy their desire, they overindulged. Many died from their gluttony. (See Numbers 11:31–34.)

God often described the promised land to the Israelites in terms of its food:

> *A land of wheat and barley, of vines and fig trees and pomegranates, a land of olive oil and honey; a land in which you will eat bread without scarcity, in which you will lack nothing.*
>
> (Deuteronomy 8:8–9)

In the temptation of Christ in the wilderness, Satan said, *"If You are the Son of God, command that these stones become bread"* (Matthew 4:3).

Food has always played a powerful role in our lives. People's lives have become unmanageable and ruinous because of their addiction to eating. Now recognizing it as a serious health problem, the American Psychiatric Association has named this unnatural and destructive attachment to food "compulsive overeating" and "bulimia." Scripture simply calls it "gluttony."

The Overeater's Syndromes

Nearly all of us have overindulged at some time in our lives. Why do we overeat? Here are just a few reasons:

• *The clean plate syndrome:* Many of us grew up eating everything on our plates because our parents reminded us of the starving people in other nations.

• *The boredom syndrome:* When we have nothing else to do, we raid the refrigerator or head for the closest fast-food restaurant to lift us out of the doldrums.

• *The grazing syndrome:* Because food always seems to be within reach, we tend to eat anytime and anywhere.

• *The unconsciousness syndrome:* We are hardly aware of what we're eating or how much or how often. We don't even know when we are full and will eat until abdominal pain stops us.

• *The blame-it-on-others syndrome:* We have a thousand reasons for blaming why we're eating on other people. We can always say, "If you weren't such a great cook..." or "If you just hadn't put it in front of me..." or "If you just hadn't offered me the chocolate...."

• *The blame-it-on-misfortune syndrome:* We also have a thousand reasons for blaming why we are eating on our misfortune. We can always say, "If only I had enough love, more money, and a good figure." Or we can say, "If only I had gotten that appointment, that job, or that promotion."

This list of syndromes could fill a whole book. Eating disorders are destroying people's lives physically, emotionally, mentally, and spiritually. The American Medical Association now recognizes eating disorders as a full-fledged disease—just like alcoholism.

Poisoning Ourselves

The average American annually eats three to five pounds of the more than 10,000 different chemicals injected into processed, preserved, and artificially colored and flavored foods. One piece of commercial fruit pie alone may contain dozens of different chemicals.

These foreign substances were never meant to enter the body. They are all anti-vital and anti-life! These poisons and carcinogens set the stage for acute and chronic disease. Since the body recognizes these counterfeit foods as poison and not as food, they are treated as such. A healthy body has enough nerve energy to expel them immediately. But the typical toxic American ingests so many poisons and has so little nerve energy to eliminate them that the body simply stores the poisons. This sows the seeds of acute and chronic disease in later years.

We invariably reap what our lifestyles have sown. Harvest time comes as we approach middle and old age. The very elderly rarely suffer from colds because their bodies have lost the vitality to conduct an acute healing crisis to eliminate toxic waste. They've slipped into the low vitality that comes with chronic autointoxication. When an older person dies, the ultimate cause is often pneumonia. The body had reached its deadly, toxic overload stage. The body was so enervated and toxic that the immune system could no longer detoxify the onslaught of bodily-created and ingested toxins. Toxin conquers and life ends.

We've neglected natural healing for too long. Taking pills to numb the pain is a quick fix, but we also disconnect the warning signals that something is wrong. Masking symptoms with drugs only accelerates the inflammation of the tissue while acute and chronic disease builds.

In advanced cases of chronic, degenerative disease, so much tissue damage has occurred that the body cannot fully restore itself to health, even with fasting.

Yet given the ideal conditions for health and given a fast followed by strict adherence to God's natural foods, the body can at least arrest the degeneration. At best, a fast will restore some of the damaged tissue to a level of functional integrity.

Breaking Free from Food's Grasp

My intention has not been to add any more of a burden to those who already feel guilty about their eating habits or their weight. I only want to point out the power that food holds over us. The apostle Paul said that while all things are lawful, not everything is helpful. He further declared, *"I will not be brought under the power of any"* (1 Corinthians 6:12). Before I can state a case for physical healing and fasting, I must make a case for the power of too much food and the wrong kinds of foods. We must become aware of Satan's strong downward pull to sedate ourselves, reward ourselves, escape ourselves, sicken ourselves, and destroy ourselves with the wrong foods in the wrong amounts!

When most people first hear about fasting for physical healing, they hesitate. "Who, me? Fast?" I understand. The idea of fasting is hard to accept. Without proper information, it's not easy to understand why God would ask His people to do it. Once fully informed, however, you will reap the blessing and benefits of fasting.

After my personal experience, study, and discussions with Christians around the world, I'm convinced that fasting requires the utmost in discipline. Because it has been out of vogue for a long time, we've fallen into eating habits that we don't want to change.

I can't promise that fasting will be easy. Self-discipline seldom is. But to those who sincerely want God's best in life, we owe it to ourselves to at least investigate the discipline of fasting. The next chapter describes another time I received healing for a serious physical condition through fasting. You'll also learn some principles of faith and fasting that I discovered.

Ten

Faith and Fasting

Several months before my twenty-one day fast in which the Lord healed me of rheumatoid vasculitis, I suffered with angina pectoris. Like many people approaching middle-age, I began to experience strange pains in my chest that extended into my neck and down my left arm. The crushing sensation in my chest alarmed me. I had to sleep propped up in bed with two or three pillows for support to make breathing easier.

Still the pains and gasping for air continued. Every night I awakened with a start. One night, even though still half asleep, I threw my legs and feet over the side of the bed and sat up as straight as possible. In a state of panic, I called, “Elmer!”

“Huh? What’s wrong?” he answered, groggy with sleep.

“My left arm and leg are numb,” I whispered in astonishment. Elmer massaged both my arm and leg until the feeling gradually returned.

A few nights later, the same thing happened, except my pelvic area also went numb. Instead of waking

Elmer, I determined to help myself. I prayed silently. Mustering all my faith and concentration, I finally maneuvered myself so that I could stand. I felt no pain. Worse yet, I felt nothing. I sat quietly and forced myself to swing my left leg. With my right hand I massaged my left arm. As feeling returned, I stood and forced myself to walk slowly across the room.

This became almost a nightly pattern. Sometimes I felt so tired that I gave up, crawled back into bed, and fell asleep with parts of my body still numb. By morning the numbness disappeared, and I could continue my normal routine.

My problem crescendoed to a frightening stage during Thanksgiving and Christmas. The holidays had been marvelous with the presence of family, friends, and special holiday food. But, as I learned later, I had experienced too much of the good life, mainly from eating too many rich foods.

The doctor diagnosed my symptoms as angina pectoris. He lectured me, explaining the kind of pain I could expect from then on. When the anginal pain hit, especially after a heavy meal, I sought relief by placing a small nitroglycerin tablet under my tongue.

"What's the cure for this?" I asked my doctor. "Surgery?"

He shook his head. "I'm sorry, Mrs. Bueno. There is no cure for angina. We can arrest it. If you take good care of yourself, you'll have a minimal amount of pain, but…."

I struggled with his pronouncement for a long time. Should I accept it? I wondered. After all, as we grow older, the body tends to wear out. Yet I knew that I had brought this condition upon myself because of my foolish habits: wrong food, not enough exercise, overwork, and not enough rest and sleep. I had been burning the candle at both ends. My symptoms forced me to realize I simply was not a superwoman and that I must strive to reverse this condition.

My First Therapeutic Fast

I had read enough about natural healing to know that serious medical problems could be alleviated through fasting. But I wrestled with the matter of faith. Did I really believe that fasting was the best answer to my physical ailment? I agreed with Dr. Shelton and others who had written on the subject. But did I have faith that it would work for me? After a protracted time of prayer, I believed God would honor my plea if I went on an absolute fast. This would be my very first therapeutic fast.

To get away from all the distractions, I went to a health spa in Florida. I had fasted many times for spiritual reasons, but this was my first therapeutic fast. My studies had given me a lot of head knowledge on fasting, but through this fast I wanted to experience physical healing.

This law of health operates in all living organisms: wherever there is life, the law of healing is constantly at work. I firmly believe this principle. Given the ideal conditions for health, living organisms always work toward restoration. Sickness occurs because we don't provide these ideal conditions and we violate the laws of life. Fasting, proper diet, and healthful lifestyles can reverse sickness and disease.

Now I had the opportunity to prove this principle in my own body. I had fasted on several occasions, missing only a meal or two. Occasionally I went for one or two days. These short fasts allowed me to maintain my heavy work schedule. This time I decided to do it differently: I would fast for a totally different reason, and I would fast for a full fourteen days, taking only water.

With such a serious heart and circulation condition, I knew better than to embark on an extended fast without proper supervision. Here at the spa, fasting experts observed me. These fine, dedicated practitioners had fasted thousands of people. They knew how to give just the kind of support I needed. With their help, and the information I had gathered in my own studies, I knew what to expect.

During my fast, I experienced a few healing crises. It would have been strange had these not occurred. Some days I was unable to leave my bed. My extreme weakness, pain, and the sometimes accelerated heartbeat let me know that my body was receiving deep rest and was the recipient of its own self-healing and self-cleansing efforts. Although they were unpleasant, I accepted these as positive signs, showing me that the healing process was in full force. On other days, I found energy to sunbathe by the pool and even sit and listen to the informative lectures on health in the evening.

"I'm Free of Pain!"

On the fifteenth day of my fast, the sun warmed my entire room. I quietly dressed for my morning walk. With my Bible and reading glasses in hand and being careful not to awaken anyone, I slipped out of the small dorm and walked into the lush, organic gardens.

The sun's rays pushed their way through the leaves of the trees, dimming the shadows along the lane that cut through the tropical garden. I strolled over the little wooden bridge that crossed one of the waterways.

When I arrived at my favorite spot near the water, I settled on a cement bench beneath the grapefruit trees. Opening my Bible, I began to read. This was a special morning—a time of accomplishment and thanksgiving. I had put my faith to the test by coming to this spa for a two-week fast. With their limited knowledge in fasting, my doctors had discouraged my coming. Despite the warnings of some of my well-meaning but misinformed friends and relatives, I had come. They were all certain that I would completely ruin my health.

"If they could only see me now!" I shouted skyward. I was free of chest pain and panic. I could sleep the whole night through without experiencing numbness in my arm and leg. I needed no extra pillows in order to sleep. I breathed easily, and my circulation felt perfect. And I was twenty-two pounds lighter. What more could you ask for in just fourteen days?

I had done my part, and God had come through with His part. There is no cure for angina pectoris. My mother suffered with it for years. Medication gives only temporary relief. The impossible had turned to possible with fasting and prayer. I felt as if God had given me a new body through prayer and fasting. My healing was a true miracle, and I wanted to sit on that bench for the next two weeks just praising God and giving thanks to Jesus.

I glanced at my watch, surprised that time had passed so quickly. It was time to break my fast. On my way to the dining room, I stopped at the kitchen for my fast-breaking meal. I had my choice of an orange or a grapefruit, and I could have only one piece. I selected one of Florida's juicy oranges. The director instructed me to take a full hour to eat the orange. I wondered if I could make it last that long.

I slowly peeled the orange, enjoying its pungency. After pulling it apart and loosening one section, I put a small piece into my mouth, savoring my first bite of food in two weeks. Never had an orange tasted so good. This was the kind of food that would preserve my health. Immediately my heart overflowed with thanksgiving. God had healed me during the fast, and now I was enjoying His ideal food to stay in His healing graces. All I had to do was live in obedience to His natural laws.

Many years have passed since my fourteen-day fast. I still have no signs of angina pectoris. I'm becoming more nutritionally aware all the time. I'll eat a piece of pie or enjoy a full-course meal, but I try to gauge it so my enjoyment doesn't become overindulgence. By God's grace, I'm in control of my appetite—and I love it.

All Healing Comes from God

I had believed in divine healing long before God removed my angina pain during this prolonged fast. God's healing power had touched my body on many occasions. Sometimes I've had to meet God halfway, stepping out in faith. You may also have to add corresponding actions to your faith. Remember that *"faith without works is dead"* (James 2:20).

After triumphing over such a debilitating condition, I was convinced of one truth: all healing comes from God. Sometimes He gives it to us in a surprise package. Other times He heals because He honors our faith. Our bodies often heal themselves because we obey God's physiological laws of life. Because God created the body to constantly heal itself, the care we give it determines the health we enjoy.

People often want immediate healing with no strings attached. We often shun going on a special diet, or disciplining ourselves in any way, in order to receive healing. With the possibility of a divine touch from God, believers sometimes shirk their own God-given responsibility.

Now I know that it takes less effort to accept the truth, apply it daily, and live in divine health. Sometimes people continue in health-destroying indulgences while they patiently wait for something that never happens. Will you wait for a miraculous experience or the special touch from a faith healer when you can actually do something about your condition? With the same ease that we turn on the TV, we want effortless, instantaneous, glorious healing. The lesser the effort, the more attractive the plan.

Miraculous healings do occur. I have come to believe, however, that God gradually releases His healing power more often as people conscientiously apply healthful living practices. This way believers learn to stretch their faith over long periods of time until healing is complete.

Health Is Our Own Responsibility

How did I learn this principle? On a warm spring day, about three years before my healing fast, Elmer and

I were comfortably seated in our air-conditioned car, purring along the interstate through California's Mojave Desert. Raising my voice above the humming of the engine, I read from a book on fasting that we had bought at a health food store just before leaving home. We were headed to Tecopa Hot Springs for a few days to soak in the sun and bathe in Tecopa's natural mineral waters. We also planned to fast.

"Man's health is his own responsibility," I read aloud. My eyes automatically returned to reread that sentence. I repeated it. "Man's health is his own responsibility." I leaned my head back against the cushioned car seat to think about it.

Noticing my silence, Elmer asked, "What's wrong?"

With the book still open on my lap and with my eyes closed, I said it again. "Man's health is his own responsibility! That's a new thought for me," I said. "I'm sure I've heard it before, but right now I accept it as true for my own health."

I hadn't believed that my actions would make a significant difference in my health. I had always thought, "This is my health. Good or bad, it's all a matter of chance." I had learned to deal with whatever came my way. If I became ill, I could turn to God and the doctors to make the necessary corrections. Preventive health care never struck me as being my responsibility or within my control.

I opened my eyes as I grasped the implications of that simple sentence. "For years, Elmer, I've been putting the blame for my poor health everywhere else. I blamed my mother for my bad teeth because she was ill when she carried me. A calcium deficiency must have caused all those cavities, because the dentist had filled every tooth by the time I was six. It had been the doctor's fault for not diagnosing my illness correctly. I blamed the medication when it didn't work. It was your fault, Elmer, for scheduling too much work and expecting me to keep up the pace. And the children's demands often frazzled my nerves. I never blamed myself for a moment of ill health!"

Like the dazzling sun dawning on a dark desert, new thoughts streamed into my mind. "By placing responsibility elsewhere, I've escaped all feelings of guilt for all my illnesses all my life!" That one sentence brought me face-to-face with my lifetime of denial and blame. "I'm the only person who is responsible for my own health. No one else."

As the car sped along, Elmer sat in silence and listened. I recounted all the memories of bad health and their consequent miseries in my life. I had been quite an expert in shifting responsibility and laying blame everywhere else.

Elmer listened, nodding his head and agreeing with every word. At the conclusion of my monologue, he said softly, "That's something I've been trying to tell you all these years." I didn't resent his words, and he hadn't said them to hurt me. Besides, I needed to hear them. Elmer had been trying for years to get through to me.

Before now, I hadn't realized that God never intended to do everything for us. Even after Adam and Eve showed their lack of responsibility, God gave them more opportunities to learn it. He commissioned them to till the land and subdue the animals. God could have thrown up His hands at their utter helplessness and decided to let them be irresponsible children forever. Instead, He gave the couple opportunities to mature by developing their responsibility.

Applying this idea of responsibility to our own health, I realized that God created our bodies with the ability to heal ourselves. While driving through the desert that day, I finally realized that I had failed to supply my body with the right conditions for healing itself.

At that moment, God handed me the key to overcome my own self-inflicted, poor health. God gave me the knowledge and power to become healthy once and for all. I had previously settled for much less than vibrant, glowing health.

"Yes, Elmer, I'm the one who salts my food too much, no matter how many times you ask me not to." I had never acknowledged that before. "Yes, Elmer, now I know that I am the one who prefers the chips and dip over fresh fruit. I am the one who drinks too much coffee. It's my fault when I refuse your cheery invitation to join you in walking a mile. Nobody else manages my schedule but me. I'm the one who hasn't learned to simply say no. And I'm the one who willingly takes on more than I can handle."

I knew that I had to face the truth. I was conducting my own encounter group, speaking the truth no matter how much it hurt. Yes, I was guilty of destroying my own health. My attitude had been, "Whatever will be, will be." I had been out of control, and my irresponsibility had robbed me of vibrant health. Worse yet, I had expected God to make me healthy with His healing touch.

Overwhelmed with this thought, I wondered in amazement, "Where was my thinking all these years? Why hasn't this truth penetrated my brain until now?" Analyzing my past behavior in this light, I marveled, "I sincerely saw myself as a victim of my unavoidable heredity and uncontrollable circumstances."

That illogical, irresponsible thinking had thrown my gears into reverse while I waited for God's big miracles. I claimed my healings by faith like a good, Bible-believing Christian. I had experienced healing several times, two of them quite spectacular. "God just has mercy on us sometimes," I continued, "even when we fail to realize the confidence He has placed in us to care for this magnificent body."

Seeing the road sign pointing to Tecopa Hot Springs, we turned right and headed east. Pulling into the little familiar town, my thoughts went back to my teenage years. I mused, "If Mother were alive, she would have loved to join us today and hear me discuss health issues."

Mother had tried to regain her failing health. She came to these same hot, soothing mineral waters and frequented the health food stores. Yet she never did find the healing secrets for which she searched. I remembered teasing her once, calling her "one of those health nuts."

"You just wait," she had admonished me. "A few years from now when you no longer have youth on your side, you'll be doing the same things."

Now, nearly twenty-five years later, I traveled a long distance to bathe in Tecopa's hot, soothing mineral waters. We certainly had been visiting lots of health food stores lately. As I related my reminiscing to Elmer, I smiled a wry, little smile. "You know something? Mama was right!" Mama had tried to explain to me several times, but I had not been ready to listen.

Making a Change

How can we alter destructive lifestyle habits? First, we must be ready to accept God's healing message. Otherwise, we don't hear it, no matter how convincingly others speak. It's just like salvation. The soil has to be fertile before the seed can lodge there and grow.

When the angina pectoris first started bothering me, I knew God wanted me to fast for my physical healing. But I needed time before I willingly disciplined myself in that way. Gradually, I knew God would heal me if I stepped out in faith and fasted.

We can't force the disciplines of fasting, proper nutrition, and healthful living practices on others. Those with whom we share must be ready, receptive, and willing to learn. Such a person may be healthy and simply want more of God's abundance, or he may be very sick and desperate. Some are willing to listen only because they've exhausted all the quick-fix schemes and need a solution.

A friend who reviewed my first draft of this book commented, "Today, we're already too burdened with failure. Why load people down with more condemnation that tells them there's something else they've done wrong?"

I answered her by sharing that none of us changes until a crisis occurs. Only when we've hit a critical time in our lives will we wholeheartedly seek to change.

After all, why should we want to change if were already doing everything right? Why discipline ourselves if everything is just fine as we travel the easy, soft way in life? Why change when we think we can't alter our destiny? Why change what we're doing when it's everyone else's fault, anyway?

Americans should look at the cause of our physical problems. Why is our country thirty-seventh on the list of the healthiest countries? Many primitive areas of the world rank far ahead of us. Admitting we're on the wrong track gives us the incentive for constructive change.

We Reap What We Sow

Not long ago, two people seated near me were discussing caffeine and its adverse effects. One man wasn't convinced that caffeine was a harmful drug. He explained that as long as he wasn't sure, he was free to indulge. "God won't hold me responsible or allow me to suffer any ill effects if I'm doing it in innocence," he asserted. I answered him with the next point.

God's natural laws don't change to accommodate uninformed minds. As I listened to that discussion on caffeine, I thought of the verse, *"My people are destroyed for lack of knowledge"* (Hosea 4:6). Because of the depth of our addictions, we often don't want to have that knowledge, either.

We can't expect the police not to give us traffic tickets just because we were unaware of the speed limit and we had exceeded it by ten miles per hour. Ignorance doesn't free us from the penalty of breaking the laws. We still have to suffer the consequences of our irresponsibility, whether we act in ignorance or in full knowledge of the deed. There is a penalty, all the same.

I'm reminded of a rude little trick we used as kids. Sometimes the only way we felt we could win an argument with a playmate was to plug our ears with our fingers, close our eyes, and shout, "I can't hear you!" This brought the discussion to a halt, leaving the other kid frustrated and angry because we refused to listen to his side of the argument. Even as adults, we sometimes resort to playing kids' games. We close our eyes, plug our ears, and shout, hoping that what we don't want to hear will go away.

Refusing to hear God's truth does not change the facts. We reap what we sow. God's natural laws also apply to our health. The care we give to our bodies brings about corresponding results. We need to educate ourselves and gain whatever knowledge is available.

For some people, giving up coffee or anything that causes withdrawal symptoms is just too great a sacrifice. When we decide to indulge, we should be ready to pay the price without complaining. We have made the choice. If the symptoms of toxemia and tissue degeneration appear, we have no right to blame anyone but ourselves. We can't ignore all the warnings, live carelessly, and destroy our bodies while expecting God to keep us in divine health.

Get to the Source

Too often we treat the symptoms instead of removing the cause. We scream at the pain, but the pain only signals that we have violated a natural law. It solves nothing. A wise man once said, "We must extinguish the fire, not just silence the siren." Instead of giving the body ideal conditions for health, we ignore its call for help. As a result, our actions and attitudes insult the wisdom of our human bodies.

Perhaps our overeating causes indigestion. We drink too much coffee, and it triggers uncomfortable heart palpitations. We exhaust our bodies with too many stressful hours of work and not enough rest. We overtax our human capabilities and then complain when our bodies demand rest.

Remember, all these seemingly slight indiscretions in health add up. They drain the body of its precious nerve energy supply, and they add to the toxic buildup of endogenous and exogenous wastes. This sets the stage for future acute and chronic life-threatening disease.

Consider the man who suffers from lung cancer and still puffs away on his cigarettes. He may pray diligently and even believe that God will heal him. If that sounds absurd (and it is), aren't we doing the same thing when we knowingly abuse our bodies and expect God to heal us? Often believers rationalize their self-destructive, pleasure-padded lifestyles by believing that "God will heal me in His time."

If we occasionally relapse into the wrong living practices, then we can repent, stop indulging ourselves, and ask God to remove the heart palpitations and the coffee cravings. They'll probably dissipate on their own because we've removed the cause by ceasing the indulgence. When we stop overeating and eating unhealthy foods, we automatically eliminate problems with indigestion. If we allow our bodies proper rest, we won't feel tired. When we stop smoking, we can ask God to remove the cancer. When we do our part, then we can expect God to do His.

Recognize Your Adversary

Satan always takes advantage of our weaknesses. We open ourselves to Satan's disease attacks when we carelessly indulge in the pleasures of wrong living practices. Satan will never miss an opportunity to destroy. We must assume responsibility for our own health. Until we take charge in that way, we can't properly activate our faith.

God has given all believers authority over Satan and his wiles. This authority enables overcomers to rebuke Satan's attacks. God offers us this victory through His authority. But living in wanton violation of and disobedience to His natural laws will nullify that authority. If we persist in breaking God's natural health laws, we relinquish our victory over Satan's disease attacks. If we do this, we cannot expect God to answer our prayers for physical healing.

While we must be aware of the Enemy's attacks, we Christians have no right to make Satan our scapegoat. We often rebuke Satan for physical symptoms of disease in our bodies. "I'm sick, and all sickness comes from the Devil," believers explain. Satan brought sin into the world, and sin spawned our perverted desires. By indulging in gluttony or slothfulness, we experience a feeling of malaise and then actual disease. Our actions, which we need to label as sin, allow Satan's work to take place in our lives.

Satan preys on us, tempts us, bombards us, obstructs us, and tricks us with counterfeits and surprise attacks.

These harassments sometimes seem innocuous and purely circumstantial. But he intends to destroy us, nevertheless. The Bible warns us,

> *We do not wrestle against flesh and blood, but against principalities, against powers, against the rulers of the darkness of this age, against spiritual hosts of wickedness in the heavenly places.* (Ephesians 6:12)

By placing our wrongdoing solely on Satan's shoulders, we do exactly what he wants. As long as we absolve ourselves of personal responsibility for our health, we will never seek change. When the consequences of wrong living come, we get wrapped up in denial by rebuking Satan. Doing that inevitably robs us of our God-given victory in Christ.

Obedience Takes Effort

Changing destructive lifestyle patterns means we have to break old habits and create new ones. The word *habit* originated from the word *costume,* and it originally referred to the habit of nuns. Habits are behavior patterns we put on or take off. If our heart muscles need to bc strengthened and if jogging three times per week will produce the results, we have a responsibility to put on the jogging habit. If sugar causes our nerves to be on edge, we need to take off the sugar habit.

But taking off the habit is easier said than done. A dear Christian woman who suffers from rheumatoid arthritis is growing progressively worse. She's been looking for the magic pill and waiting for the divine touch. She has dozens of prescription drugs, over-the-counter medicines, and countless bottles of potions suggested by doctors and friends.

Medicine bottles line her cupboard shelves. She's always the first one in the healing line for prayer at church!

By the way, there is no medical cure for rheumatoid arthritis. The doctors usually tell their patients, "You must learn to live with it." At best, doctors offer drugs that give temporary relief but bring horrible side effects.

One day I mentioned that her arthritis could be healed, or at least greatly controlled, by fasting and a proper diet. When I made my suggestion, her husband sadly replied, "Oh, she knows all that, but she just won't do it."

As they walked away, I kept thinking, *"Faith without works is dead"* (James 2:26). Divine healing is a gift; but when people knowingly abuse their bodies, they cannot rightfully expect God's gift of healing. *"Therefore, to him who knows to do good and does not do it, to him it is sin"* (James 4:17).

We can activate faith by doing what is in our own power. This is a positive step toward health. We can employ fasting for health maintenance, for minor acute flare-ups, or for life-threatening disease. But we won't be motivated unless our faith has corresponding actions.

What can I do to strengthen my failing faith? The answer lies within the pages of this book. Put action to that faith by developing correct living habits. Diligently apply them. These life-giving ingredients recharge our faith. God created our bodies to heal themselves. We can pray and fast in faith, knowing that God will bring healing to us.

Eleven

The Spiritual Fast

Fasting unto the Lord, sometimes called the spiritual or religious fast, is conducted primarily for spiritual benefit. The spiritual fast, which can be an individual or a proclaimed fast, is a total, absolute, or partial fast of any duration. God may lead you to conduct a total fast for one to three days, or you may undertake an absolute or partial fast for several weeks. This can be a regularly practiced form of worship. You may also want to fast unto the Lord at the prompting of the Holy Spirit with a specific spiritual goal, need, or request in mind.

In Bible times, people often fasted unto the Lord as a memorial or to commemorate a certain event in history. The Jews fasted each year on the Day of Atonement. Another example of this is Purim, in memory of the fast proclaimed by Esther to the Jewish people—the fast that saved their lives.

A spiritual fast can be conducted almost any place and time, as long as the faster understands the significance of fasting unto the Lord. We can undertake a spiritual fast even while continuing our work and church activities. This is one of the differences between the therapeutic and the spiritual fast. Fasting for physical healing requires bed rest so that the body can replenish its nerve energy supply, detoxify itself, and repair unhealthy tissues. If you're already healthy when you undertake a spiritual fast, you don't need urgent bed rest. The faster may continue his daily routine as his energy levels allow.

Many Christians have shared amazing stories of how they have conducted their own spiritual fasts. A Canadian butcher never missed a day of work while conducting a forty-day absolute fast. He was able to carry large sides of beef and never had to slow his pace because of weakness. He also received the spiritual benefit he was seeking. (Such an extended fast could harm the body of an inexperienced faster. Do not fast for long periods of time on your first attempt.)

Today, believers seldom fast at all. The spiritual fast of short duration—from one meal to a few days—is the only kind of fasting most Christians practice. As you begin to fast unto the Lord at the leading of the Holy Spirit, we recommend that you start with a fast of shorter duration. If you must handle your normal work and family responsibilities, you may want to try the partial fast.

What Is a Consecration Fast?

The most serious of all spiritual fasts, the consecration fast, is an absolute fast of extended duration undertaken for highly personal reasons. The consecration fast differs greatly from a spiritual fast such as the one the Canadian butcher undertook. During the consecration fast, the individual takes only water—usually for many days—as he fully devotes himself to God. Historically, the individual fasted for forty days. Today, people may fast for longer periods of time, or to completion when hunger returns. The consecration fast usually lasts much longer than the more common spiritual fast.

Christians often undertake a spiritual fast for answers to specific prayer requests. A consecration fast, however, is a monumental act of supplication in which our desires, our goals, and our very lives are aligned with God's purposes. A consecrated fast prepares us to fulfill God's plan, not our own selfish ambitions.

The best way to appreciate the consecration fast is to reflect on Jesus' forty-day fast in the wilderness. He set Himself apart from others and sought God to learn His purpose on earth. Total surrender to God becomes the sole purpose of the consecration fast. After being led by the Holy Spirit into the wilderness to fast, Jesus *"returned in the power of the Spirit to Galilee, and news of Him went out through all the surrounding region"* (Luke 4:14). The Gospels record the works of power that flowed through this yielded vessel. Jesus' example should encourage us to fast, too.

Before undertaking the consecration fast, prayerfully consider these nine basic questions:

1. Am I in good health?
2. Can I find a private place for fasting?
3. Can I stop working while I fast?
4. Can I fast for no special request—just to worship?
5. Will fasting make me more spiritual?
6. Will fasting strengthen my ability to minister to others?

7. Will the Holy Spirit lead me into the consecration fast?
8. What should I expect to receive from God while fasting?
9. What if I can't find time for the consecration fast?

Let's look at each consideration in more detail. As you prayerfully weigh the costs and benefits of the consecration fast, God will make His will increasingly clear to you.

Am I in Good Health?

We can only assume that Jesus entered His fast in good health. After all, He had kept the dietary and hygienic laws of Moses. He enjoyed fresh air and exercise. Jesus didn't succumb to the gamut of negative emotions such as guilt, worry, and fear that cause illness. We can safely assume that Jesus entered His consecration fast in excellent health, ready to receive the fullest spiritual benefit possible.

If you're in good health, you can undertake the consecration fast. If you suffer from acute or chronic illness, you'll need to fast for therapeutic reasons, preferably under supervision. After you've regained your health, your nerve energy is high, and you've replenished your reserves through a period of eating wholesome foods, then you can consider the consecration fast. If the individual can't pray and read the Bible because of physical discomforts that come with a healing crisis, he should postpone the consecration fast until he regains his health and his reserves are high.

One minister attended our fasting class at Christian Retreat in Bradenton, Florida. He was so enthusiastic about the morning classes that he always sat in the front row with a pencil and pad in hand and a Bible at his side. On the final morning of the seminar, he shared his story:

> Not long ago, I planned a consecration fast. I instructed my wife not to bother me and not to let anyone know my whereabouts. I took a stack of Bibles and study books, shut myself away in one of the rooms at the church, and began my ten-day fast. But I couldn't read a line. All I could do was sleep. Satan himself seemed to oppose me, but I just couldn't overcome my drowsiness. I couldn't pray or study, so I gave up after only two days.

This minister made three mistakes in conducting his fast. First, he had closed himself up in a room. Yes, he needed privacy, but he probably needed to walk outdoors, too. This renews the mind and helps to increase alertness, peace, and resolve to continue fasting.

Second, the desire to sleep is natural, especially during the first few days of a fast. Don't view this as satanic. If the faster has been overworked before the fast, this is a natural response. The body is detoxifying and restoring nerve energy. Later in the fast, a newfound alertness will occur. The minister needed to sleep as often as it came upon him.

Third, the minister could have prepared for the consecration fast by conducting a series of short therapeutic fasts followed by eating wholesome, natural foods. This regimen would have alleviated any health problems so the minister could have been in fine shape for consecrating himself unto the Lord.

The consecration fast loses its purpose when fasters become concerned about detoxification symptoms and each healing crisis that occurs in their bodies. This moves them into the category of the therapeutic faster whose symptoms and pain need proper supervision. To receive the greatest benefit from the consecration fast, we must undertake it in reasonably good health. Only then can we devote ourselves to prayer and supplication.

Can I Find a Private Place?

Most of us who consider any kind of prolonged fasting usually find this consideration the hardest to execute. Picking the spot is not as difficult as finding oneself alone with God for prolonged periods of time. We discover that we are not as close to the Lord as we had believed.

Why do people experience such stark loneliness while fasting unto the Lord? We've spent too much time gratifying our senses and indulging our desires in the world. We've never learned how to be alone with God for long periods of time. Few of our spiritual leaders actually do it, and we have no firsthand experience in praying without ceasing.

For the greatest spiritual benefits, we need to conduct our consecration fast away from the crowds. We should spend as much time as possible in seclusion, resting in the Lord and being assured that He is with us. Not feeling His presence as intensely as during praise and worship in church doesn't mean we are alienated from Him. We need to be still, to listen to the soft voice of the Holy Spirit, and to accept the peace that comes with the hours of prayer and fasting.

Enjoying the stillness of God's presence comes easily for me. I spend entire days completely alone with the Lord. I mature in my faith more when I can be alone with Jesus. I wrote the first draft of this book while I was alone in a comfortable but isolated spot in Death Valley, California. The solitude, peace, and quiet secured in the desert led me to report to a friend, "This is better than Valium any day!"

I learned to enjoy solitude when I was an only child and had to amuse myself for hours. Several times, my illness forced me to be alone. Rheumatic fever confined me to bed for two years of my childhood. I spent much of that time in a hospital, away from my parents. Learning to be alone with God became a way of life at an early age. When fasting became a part of my life, I was prepared to enjoy the quiet, long hours in fellowship with God.

Knowing that this is not the case for most Christians, I encourage you to persevere. The boredom and frustration inherent in fasting may be the most formidable barrier to conquer. Stimulation and excitement fill our lives. The American way of life revolves around action and diversion. How can we learn to cultivate stillness? When we practice the discipline of solitude, we learn to enjoy it. Only then can we reap great benefits from it.

When I counsel people who encounter loneliness during fasting, I urge them, "You'll have to be a little more flexible in this area. God sees your heart and knows what you can and can't do." I want to make it clear that everyone should not necessarily be alone 100 percent of the time, isolated in the desert somewhere. Simple privacy, however, is important.

Elmer once undertook a twenty-one day consecration fast. He changed his routine from office work and travel to time working alone in the garden. He prays better outside than in a room. In the garden he found hours of seclusion, and he didn't need to leave home. Each of us must consider our own situation and decide what will work best for us.

In considering this matter of privacy, look at the prophet Daniel shortly after his fast. God wanted Daniel alone, but He found him in the company of several other men. God's presence overwhelmed Daniel's friends and *"a great terror fell upon them, so that they fled to hide themselves"* (Daniel 10:7). Daniel didn't run in fear. His heart had been spiritually seasoned with his twenty-one day fast. Daniel reported, *"Therefore I was left alone when I saw this great vision"* (verse 8).

Look at the example of other great men of the Bible who learned to spend time alone with God and profited immeasurably from their experiences:

- Abraham lived alone upon the heights, but Lot chose to live among the people in Sodom. (See Genesis 13:12.)

- Moses was skilled in all the wisdom of Egypt, yet he spent forty years alone in the wilderness. (See Acts 7:22–30.)

- Paul, a great scholar, had the highest education possible in his day by studying under the great Gamaliel; yet after his conversion he went into Arabia to be alone with God. (See Galatians 1:15–17.)

• Jesus spent time alone in the wilderness with God in preparation for His ministry. (See Matthew 4:1–2.)

God will speak to us when He has our undivided attention. Through the consecration fast we develop such a powerful relationship with God that the soul learns to depend on its own faith, rather than continually needing support and bolstering from others.

Can I Stop Working?

Some people combine the consecration fast with a heavy workload. Most of them wonder why their time didn't yield results. "What happened?" they innocently ask, never realizing that their attention had been divided between God and the world the whole time. Here are several biblical answers to this question:

• When God called his people to fast on the Day of Atonement, He specifically commanded complete rest for them, their servants, and any visitor who might be passing through the country. (See Leviticus 16:29.)

• When the Israelites complained that they were fasting but saw no results, they learned that they displeased God by making their servants work. (See Isaiah 58:3.)

• When the prophet Joel proclaimed a fast, he called for a solemn assembly, and nobody works at a solemn assembly! (See Joel 2:15.)

When God leads us to begin a consecration fast, we must ask for wisdom on how best to seek our privacy for the greatest spiritual benefit. Continuing other activities will only divide the intellect from the heart, which will defeat the purpose of the consecration fast.

Can I Fast for No Specific Request?

People often ask, "Why should I fast? I don't have any special problems." We don't have to encounter special problems to fast. It isn't necessary to fast and pray for someone's special need or agonize over personal requests.

We may enter the consecration fast as a form of worship. We can wait on God, making ourselves available to do His will. In a consecrated fast we set ourselves apart from the world, from food and drink, from all earthly pleasures and sensual comforts of life. *"And* [you] *shall honor Him, not doing your own ways, nor finding your own pleasure, nor speaking your own words"* (Isaiah 58:13).

God takes glory in such a fast. He appreciates that His people take time to worship Him, asking nothing from Him in return. Isn't this a beautiful way to glorify God? By simply abstaining from food, humbling our souls, and setting worldly matters aside in an act of worship, we can please God beyond compare.

Will I Be More Spiritual?

A friend once asked, "Will I become a 'spiritual giant' if I undertake the consecration fast?" The expression on her face was both serious and innocent. We have no guarantees before we fast. This is not a bargain in which we promise to forgo food for ten days in exchange for a greater level of spirituality, power, ministry, and knowledge.

Fasters may receive a special vision or an extraordinary revelation from God. This can and does happen, but it should never be our motivation. Fasting is not the biblical equivalent of waving a magic wand to make all personal wishes come true. Fasting is the most sacred, most serious, most sacrificial way to present ourselves in total devotion to the Lord. A consecration fast is the best way to prepare ourselves to receive the fullness of God's blessings in our lives. Fasting helps us to relinquish our wills to God.

This isn't to say that we can't pray for specific requests in a consecration fast. Derek Prince, who has addressed this subject in his ministry, suggests that we write our petitions on a sheet of paper. Then he recommends that we put the list of requests away in a drawer and then pull it out and read it two weeks later, a month later, a year later. We may be amazed to see that God has answered every request!

During one fourteen-day fast, I had three specific requests. God answered all three before I completed the fast. This doesn't always happen. The answers may come much later—even years later. We cannot allow ourselves to get discouraged if we don't see immediate answers as soon as we break the fast.

The popular myth that fasting turns one into a "spiritual giant" does have some basis in reality, however. By fasting unto the Lord in the proper spirit and for a significant duration, one often becomes more aware of the presence of God. This heightened awareness prepares the Christian with a stronger direction and purpose in his life. He finds himself more ready for active service, better equipped to defeat Satan in spiritual warfare.

A Stronger Ministry?

The apostle Paul fasted to strengthen his ministry. Many of us follow Paul's teachings and examples—except when it comes to fasting. That's when we start making exceptions. Modern Christians have virtually omitted fasting from their lives. Neglecting this spiritual discipline has resulted in the diminished power that plagues our churches. God's glory is also diminished because we fail to follow in obedience. The apostle Paul was a spiritual athlete who recognized the power of fasting to strengthen his ministry. Paul remains the most noteworthy of all soulwinners in history, second only to Christ.

After His consecration fast, Jesus went to the synagogue at Capernaum and announced,

> *The Spirit of the LORD is upon Me, because He has anointed Me to preach the gospel to the poor; He has sent Me to heal the brokenhearted, to proclaim liberty to the captives and recovery of sight to the blind, to set at liberty those who are oppressed, to proclaim the acceptable year of the LORD.* (Luke 4:18–19)

Jesus then demonstrated these words by healing all kinds of disease, casting out devils, and raising the dead. Jesus not only fulfilled this prophecy from Isaiah, but He also promised that *"he who believes in Me, the works that I do he will do also; and greater works than these he will do, because I go to My Father"* (John 14:12).

Dake's Annotated Reference Bible states that none of us

> can receive greater power than Jesus, for He received the Spirit without measure. Therefore, the "greater works" could not consist of doing greater things than Christ could have done had He had the occasion to do them....Each believer can have equal power with Christ to do what He did, as well as greater things if and when the occasion requires it.[1]

This anointing we receive during the consecration fast is for ministry. God told Moses, *"You shall anoint Aaron and his sons, and consecrate them, that they may minister to me as priests"* (Exodus 30:30). Similarly, God anoints us by His Holy Spirit to minister to others as a result of our consecrated time spent with Him.

Let's examine another significant passage that illustrates the power of prayer and fasting. While Jesus took Peter, James, and John to the mountain where He was transfigured, the rest of His disciples tried to cast a demon out of a boy. When their attempts were unsuccessful, the boy's father appealed to Jesus. He rebuked the demon, and the boy was well from that hour. The disciples came to Jesus privately and asked why they couldn't cast the demon out. Jesus replied, *"This kind does not go out except by prayer and fasting"* (Matthew 17:21).

Will the Holy Spirit Lead Me?

The Holy Spirit led Jesus into the wilderness to begin His consecration fast. The Spirit will also lead us—if we want to be led. Perhaps we need to ask ourselves the following questions if we've never fasted unto the Lord for any length of time:

- Is the Spirit leading me to follow Jesus' example?
- Have I hindered the Spirit by not listening?
- Because of not understanding the importance of fasting, have I been hesitant to fast?

Most of us wouldn't entertain the idea to forgo food for an extended period of time without a special sign from God. Reading this book may be your first sign. The Spirit of God initiates the desire within us through such signs. Pray for guidance to confirm God's specific direction for your fast. Ask Him what type of fast you should undertake and how long it should be. Don't rush into a prolonged fast on your first attempt. Once we receive confirmation that the Lord is calling us to fast, we can be led by the Holy Spirit to conduct the consecration fast.

To receive that confirmation from God, we should give careful thought to each of the nine considerations in this chapter. We must prayerfully ask that the will of God would be primary in our hearts. When we have this attitude, all hesitation, doubt, and fear will vanish.

After Paul's conversion, he retreated to the Arabian Desert. (See Galatians 1:15–17.) He consecrated himself to the Lord as he readjusted his theology to incorporate Jesus. Although he was highly educated in the religious world of that day, he did not seek instruction from the recognized leaders, the obvious place for counsel. He sought a different Source in the desert.

Considering the time, the place, and the man, there is little doubt that Paul fasted when he went to Arabia. Fasting was not uncommon to him even before his conversion. In fact, it was the first thing he did after his encounter on the road to Damascus. Like Paul, we should seek refuge in privacy and consecrate our lives to do God's will.

What Will I Receive?

Most of us tend to minimize the importance of fasting unless we have been formally educated to do otherwise. After all, fasting is one of the most difficult and misunderstood of all spiritual disciplines. Furthermore, fasting is "out of style" in our overfed, fast-food times. Food grips many believers in its powerful grasp.

Yet the Bible tells us, *"The earnest expectation of the creation eagerly waits for the revealing* [manifestation] *of the sons of God"* (Romans 8:19). To manifest means to make clear or obvious. *"But the manifestation of the Spirit is given to each one for the profit of all"* (1 Corinthians 12:7). This verse refers to spiritual gifts. These manifestations or spiritual gifts are the way God reveals the truth of the Gospel. As we glorify God through fasting, these gifts are made more readily available for us to use. Let's look at that entire passage.

> *But the manifestation of the Spirit is given to each one for the profit of all: for to one is given the word of wisdom through the Spirit, to another the word of knowledge through the same Spirit, to another faith by the same Spirit, to another gifts of healings by the same Spirit, to another the working of miracles, to another prophecy,*

> *to another discerning of spirits, to another different kinds of tongues, to another the interpretation of tongues. But one and the same Spirit works all these things, distributing to each one individually as He wills. For as the body is one and has many members, but all the members of that one body, being many, are one body, so also is Christ.* (1 Corinthians 12:7–12)

The gift of healing manifested itself in Elmer's life at the conclusion of his twenty-one day consecration fast. Elmer went to visit Kathleen Morrow, who was dying of cancer. She expected to live only a few more days. Because she was hemorrhaging through the stomach, she hadn't eaten for over a week. Elmer laid his hands on her and prayed.

Kathleen Morrow testifies that as Elmer prayed, the room filled with light. After he left, she felt so much better that she asked for food. She ate and, for the first time in weeks, was able to hold the food down. Miraculously, after just two more days, she felt good enough to leave the hospital, making the trip by car from California to her home in Arizona. She said she ate all the way home. She was healed. Elmer attributes a great part of her healing to the faith that God inspired through his time of prayer and fasting.

God confirmed the apostle Paul's preaching by powerful demonstrations of the Holy Spirit. God has shown us that these messages are true by signs, wonders, and various miracles and by giving certain special abilities through the Holy Spirit to those who believe. (See Hebrews 2:4.)

According to Paul, there is no other remedy for the suffering of mankind than the manifestations of these gifts through God's people. As believers, we may impress others with the kindness of our lives and our good works, as Jesus did when He was about His Father's business. But our true ministry in the full glory and power of God will not come until we totally consecrate our lives to Him through a time of fasting and prayer. We must live by Jesus' example in all areas of our lives. Only after Jesus fasted in the wilderness did God release powerful gifts through His ministry. God bestows upon each of us one or more of His spiritual gifts. When we consecrate a fast to God, He releases these gifts through us. The Holy Spirit directs us in our daily lives to make use of them.

Unfortunately, many of us allow our spiritual gifts to lie dormant. Many of us have so little direct communication with God that we do not even recognize His special gifts. Consequently, we neither use God's gifts to serve others, nor do we work at developing them. But the Bible urges us to *"stir up the gift of God which is in* [us]*"* (2 Timothy 1:6).

Yes, God gives us the gifts, but we must do the stirring. If we have not discovered our gifts, it is because we have failed to exercise them. Someone may feel that they have lost his gift through his own spiritual neglect. This is not cause for dismay, however. It is never too late. God is always faithful and patient. Scripture affirms, *"For the gifts and the calling of God are irrevocable"* (Romans 11:29).

At first we may scarcely perceive our gifts. During the hours of fasting unto the Lord, that which we but dimly perceive starts to be revealed. As the world fades away, the Holy Spirit brightens our spiritual lives.

God begins to reveal His unique plan for us. As we execute His plan in our daily lives, we find—to our utter delight—the availability of His gifts. God imparts talents we never knew we had to be used to serve others, to take care of His world, and to glorify Him! This is the greatest single joy to the Christian: to know that we're serving Him to the best of our ability and in accord with His plan for us!

In all my years and travels, working with people who fast unto the Lord, I have yet to recall anyone who did not realize vast spiritual benefit from having given themselves over to an extended consecration fast.

What If I Can't Find Time?

Finding the time for fasting may require effort. We may need someone to care for the children, someone to handle the phone messages, another to run the office. Yet if the desires are strong enough, God will provide.

Why not use vacation time for fasting? Our son, Chris, planned a three-day fast. He went about it methodically. First, he made sure someone took his place at the office. He decided where to go and phoned for reservations. He spent his precious fasting and prayer time in a little cabin in the mountains—undisturbed, alone, and in fellowship with God.

If this book has inspired you to consecrate some time for fasting but you don't have many available days, then take what time you do have and begin your new adventure of fasting. Don't think you can't fast just because you don't have time to conduct the consecration fast. When getting away isn't possible, why not compromise by fasting one or two meals and spending a few hours in solitude? We don't have to have the perfect setting to go on a fast. If that were so, no one would ever fast at all! Scripture admonishes us that *"if you wait for perfect conditions, you will never get anything done"* (Ecclesiastes 11:4 TLB).

Whether you consecrate a fast unto the Lord for four days or forty, the answers to the previous nine considerations need your prayerful attention. In short, before entering into the consecration fast, whatever its duration, you need to:

1. Enter into the fast with good health.
2. Conduct the fast in as much seclusion as possible.
3. Remain open for God's spiritual objectives, rather than forcing your preconceived ideas onto this period of fasting and prayer.
4. Expect God to reveal His chosen plan for your life and to bestow upon you His spiritual gifts, which are the manifestations of His love and direction for your life.

If you do these things, fasting will be a positive experience for you. You'll soon want to embark on this discipline as a regular part of your spiritual life.

Twelve

Why Fast for Spiritual Reasons?

"Why should I undertake a spiritual fast?" Knowing little or nothing about fasting, many Christians don't fast because they have the same problem as the Israelites. They're overly concerned with their physical beings, or they're filled with superstition and fear, or their desire for food is too strong to give up even one meal. They neither know the value of the therapeutic fast nor understand the power that the spiritual fast can awaken in them.

Still, there will always be those who—even if they have the correct information in front of them—will protest. Here are some favorite rationalizations that deprive people of the power of God through fasting.

• *"I don't have the time."* I never argue with that statement. But I know that we have enough time to do what we consider important.

• *"But I just don't feel the need to fast."* This is an honest statement. Many believers who use this rationalization are simultaneously calling out for guidance and power in their lives, yet they block the most powerful avenue to effect the changes they so strongly desire. Scripture assures us that when we wait upon the Lord, we renew our strength. (See Isaiah 40:31.) Fasting unto the Lord is perhaps the most sincere form of waiting upon Him.

• *"But fasting might ruin my health."* By now you should realize this rationalization has no validity. Similar excuses I've heard include: "Fasting will damage my brain," "Fasting creates a potassium deficiency," and "Fasting eats up your muscles, destroys your stomach, and causes permanent physical disabilities." None of those statements are true, and even the slightest investigation shows evidence to the contrary.

❧

Nine Reasons to Fast unto the Lord

Throughout my years of teaching on fasting, people most frequently ask, "Why should I fast?" These earnest inquirers know many strong Christians who have never fasted a day in their lives. The pastors of their churches have never preached on fasting. In fact, their first formal introduction to the subject came through my ministry. I'm not surprised that they often ask me, "Why should I fast?"

My answer is usually in the form of a few sentences, a one-day seminar, or my sets of teaching tapes. In this book, however, I can fully answer that question. Here are nine reasons why we fast unto the Lord:

1. To combine the power of fasting with prayer for more dynamic results.
2. To become more like Christ.

3. To make a special request or achieve a specific goal.
4. To more fully praise, worship, and honor God.
5. To receive deeper insight and revelation from God.
6. To better prepare ourselves for serving God.
7. To more fully open our hearts to the hungry.
8. To intercede on behalf of the sins and weaknesses of others.
9. To develop self-discipline and show our commitment to God.

In an effort to fully appreciate each of these reasons for fasting unto the Lord, let me discuss each separately.

Pray and Fast For Dynamic Results

Without a doubt, the combination of fasting and prayer produces dynamic results. Combined prayer and fasting does what neither one nor the other could do alone. The following letter from a friend demonstrates what prayer and fasting can do.

> For over six years, I prayed for the salvation of my husband. After your seminar on fasting, I decided to try it. My first fast was a few days in February, and I thought it was in vain because I didn't see any positive results. In March, however, I fasted again but still didn't see any change.
>
> Now, two months later, I'm happy to report that my husband has given his heart to the Lord. After six years of prayer—and only four months of fasting and prayer—I now live with a Christian husband! Praise God!

Regardless of the combined power of fasting and prayer, someone nearly always asks, "But how do we know that prayer alone won't bring the answer?"

I usually answer, "Prayer alone may be enough. But how can we be sure?" If we can intensify our prayers and increase their effectiveness, shouldn't we do whatever it takes to see the answer come? If something is worthy of our prayer, isn't it also worthy of our fasting? St. Augustine aptly expressed the importance of this discipline: "Do you wish your prayer to fly toward God? Give it two wings: fasting and praying."

When the king of Nineveh proclaimed a fast after hearing Jonah's prediction of impending doom, he asked, *"Who can tell if God will turn and relent, and turn away from His fierce anger, so that we may not perish?"* (Jonah 3:9). When the city repented with prayer and fasting, God spared Nineveh.

Queen Esther called all Jews to a three-day fast so that she would receive the king's favor and avert the slaughter of her people. While the Bible makes no specific mention of prayer, we can certainly infer that they prayed as they fasted. (See Esther 4:16.) This fast brought the answers to her request.

These two biblical examples demonstrate that fasting intensifies prayer power. Fasting brings us before God in total dependency as we ask for His divine intervention. Fasting unto the Lord adds urgency to our prayers. By combining prayer and fasting, we express our utter helplessness to control difficult and desperate situations. Fasting is much more than mere abstinence from food and water. Fasting proclaims to God that we are nothing without Him. He is our strength, our fortress, our hope in times of trouble. When the Lord sees our faith demonstrated in fasting, He is pleased and hastens to bless our lives accordingly.

Becoming More like Christ

When Jesus began His public ministry, He went to the Jordan River to be baptized by John. As Jesus came out of the water, He saw the heavens open and the Spirit descended upon Him. A voice from heaven declared, *"You are My beloved Son, in whom I am well pleased"* (Mark 1:11). The Holy Spirit immediately led Jesus into the wilderness where He undertook His fast.

Christ's forty-day fast was no different for Him than it would be for you or me. At the end of His fast, Jesus hungered like any other human being. Having just completed His fast in forty days, His body was in the most purified state possible here on earth. With His body reserves used up, His hunger returned. He undoubtedly wanted food, yet He had not yet resumed eating. Christ waited for God to take care of His physical need.

The Bible does not give us a daily account of Jesus' fast. But Christ was tempted upon the completion of His fast. In answer to Satan, Jesus used the most powerful weapon at His disposal: the Word of God. While He received no special privilege because He was the Son of God, Jesus took advantage of the same resources still available to every Christian. Christ's time of fasting and prayer shows us that life consists of a higher existence and is not dependent upon bread alone (or any other material pleasure). We must live *"by every word that proceeds from the mouth of God"* (Matthew 4:4).

The New Testament urges us to become more like Christ in all that we say and do. God sent Jesus to be our role model. Jesus told us to be perfect, even as our heavenly Father is perfect. (See Matthew 5:48.) Does this mean we should emulate Christ in just some areas and not in others? Or does it mean that we should strive to become more like Christ in every area of life—including fasting unto the Lord?

Fast for a Specific Request

When people fast, they usually have a goal in mind. This could be an answered prayer, deeper spiritual understanding, physical healing, faith to perform miracles, a new ministry, or the development of spiritual gifts.

Jesus' forty-day fast gives us an example of obedience and discipline. He reaped spiritual benefits from this prolonged season of prayer and fasting. Jesus spent valuable time alone with His heavenly Father and received the greatest ministry history has ever known. In the same way, God will richly reward us for our times of prayer and fasting.

Because of His experience, Christ could teach the people about how and why to fast. He told His followers,

> *When you fast, anoint your head and wash your face, so that you do not appear to men to be fasting, but to your Father who is in the secret place; and your Father who sees in secret will reward you openly.* (Matthew 6:17–18)

These rewards are very special because they can be obtained in no other way except through prayer and fasting.

Do you remember the father who pleaded with Jesus to heal his lunatic son? (See Matthew 17:14–21.) The father had taken his son to the disciples for healing, but they could not deliver him. Jesus freed the demoniac while His disciples could not. They questioned Him privately, *"Why could we not cast it out?"* (verse 19). Jesus answered, *"Because of your unbelief....If you have faith as a mustard seed, you will say to this mountain, 'Move from here to there' and it will move; and nothing will be impossible for you"* (verse 20). The next verse makes this a reality: *"However, this kind does not go out except by prayer and fasting"* (verse 21). In other words, fasting purifies our faith to believe that anything is possible with God.

This is the clearest, most dramatic example of being granted special, specific requests through fasting unto the Lord. If we Christians would exercise the same discipline and fast unto the Lord with a right heart, then we would also receive God's exceedingly special rewards.

To Worship God

As explained in the last chapter, we glorify God by forsaking our own self-seeking, sensual, self-indulgent ways. When we fast unto the Lord, we strip away our worldly desires. We turn our lives, our minds, and our hearts over to God. Fasting is a way to praise, worship, and honor God. Scripture says,

> *And [you] shall honor Him, not doing your own ways, nor finding your own pleasure, nor speaking your own words, then you shall delight yourself in the Lord.* (Isaiah 58:13–14)

While we can fast for a specific prayer request or for our own spiritual growth, we can also fast just to draw near to God, giving Him our undivided attention. The less interference from everyday activities and worldly cares, the more we become one mind and one spirit with Him. This is an ideal way to seek God. When our attention is fully focused on God, we are sensitive to His faint promptings. God may convict us of sin, reassure us of His presence, or impart new vision for our lives. Because we've eliminated distractions, we're more open to carry out His will.

When we undertake a consecration fast, we must seek privacy. We need to be totally separated from the phone, work, the radio, television, the newspaper, even away from the responsibilities of family and friends. Under these conditions of self-imposed isolation, we can truly fast: giving up virtually everything that is of the world—especially eating—so that Jesus Christ may have our undivided attention and true worship.

Receiving Deeper Insights

Although we shouldn't fast just for the sake of receiving insights and visions, we can fast unto the Lord so that we will be more open to their occurrence. Genuine revelations have occurred throughout history Here are a few biblical examples of people who received revelations while fasting unto the Lord:

• Daniel, after his three-week fast, saw a vision. The Spirit told him what would befall the people in the latter days. Although in the company of several others, he alone saw the vision. He was also the only one who had been fasting. (See Daniel 10:2–7, 17.)

• Elijah, after a forty-day fast, learned who would succeed him as prophet and who would succeed the reigning kings of Israel and Syria. (See 1 Kings 19:8–18.)

• Moses, during his famous forty-day fast, received the Ten Commandments. (See Exodus 24:18; 34:27–28.)

• The psalmist received many wondrous psalms after times of fasting and prayer. (See Psalm 35:13; 69:10; 109:24.)

• Anna, the prophetess, *"served God with fastings and prayers night and day"* (Luke 2:37). Consequently, God revealed to her that the infant being presented in the temple was the Messiah.

• Cornelius fasted and then received divine revelation. An angel told him where to find Peter, the one who shared the Gospel with his family and friends. (See Acts 10:30–32.)

• Saul, before his conversion and calling as an apostle, traveled to Damascus to persecute Christians. Suddenly a light from heaven blinded him. He fell to the earth and heard a voice saying, *"Saul, Saul, why are you persecuting Me?"* (Acts 9:4). Saul's companions helped him into the city. He did not eat or drink for three days. (See verse 9.) After his fast, God told him in a vision that Ananias would lay hands on him to restore his sight and that he would also learn the great things he would suffer for the Lord's sake. (See verses 12–18.)

• Paul, during a fourteen-day fast, was shipwrecked on the Isle of Crete. An angel of God stood by him, revealed that he would be brought before Caesar, and told him that the lives of all his shipmates would be spared. (See Acts 27:3–34.) In his writings, Paul alluded to his many revelations. I'm convinced he experienced them because he was *"in fastings often"* (2 Corinthians 11:27).

• The prophets and teachers at Antioch were fasting and praying when the Holy Spirit separated Paul and Barnabas for a special work. During a fast at a prayer meeting, they were ordained as apostles. (See Acts 13:2–3.)

I'm not surprised that those were days of supernatural events! First-century believers frequently fasted and prayed. Visions, revelations, and deep insights commonly occurred among the people. Today, by contrast, the Christian who receives direct, divine messages is looked at with suspicion. Why should these divine promptings be so rare in modern America? God wants to communicate with His people and show Himself strong on their behalf.

Why aren't churchgoers experiencing the supernatural in their lives? Is it because fasting rarely accompanies the special services and prayer meetings that we schedule? Could it be that we keep our bellies too full, too often? Rather than taking lightly the supernatural events associated with fasting and prayer, shouldn't we be open to the God-given insights and revelations available with this discipline? Like the ancients, we can prepare for such communication with God through fasting and prayer. If more of us would fast unto the Lord, our faith and power would be released for greater miracles in our own lives.

Preparation for Service

This is why we should fast unto the Lord: to better prepare ourselves for service. The following passage of Scripture urges us to fast unto the Lord so that we may better serve. It also promises us inestimable blessings once we have fasted and been inspired to serve humanity.

> *Is it a fast that I have chosen, a day for a man to afflict his soul? Is it to bow down his head like a bulrush, and to spread out sackcloth and ashes? Would you call this a fast, and an acceptable day to the* LORD*? Is this not the fast that I have chosen: to loose the bonds of wickedness, to undo the heavy burdens, to let the oppressed go free, and that you break every yoke? Is it not to share your bread with the hungry, and that you bring to your house the poor who are cast out; when you see the naked, that you cover him, and not hide yourself from your own flesh? Then your light shall break forth like the morning, your healing shall spring forth speedily, and your righteousness shall go before you; the glory of the* LORD *shall be your rear guard. Then you shall call, and the* LORD *will answer; you shall cry, and He will say, "Here I am." If you take away the yoke from your midst, the pointing of the finger, and speaking wickedness, if you extend your soul to the hungry and satisfy the afflicted soul, then your light shall dawn in the darkness, and your darkness shall be as the noonday. The* LORD *will guide you continually, and satisfy your soul in drought, and strengthen your bones; you shall be like a watered garden,*

> *and like a spring of water, whose waters do not fail. Those from among you shall build the old waste places; you shall raise up the foundations of many generations; and you shall be called the Repairer of the Breach, the Restorer of Streets to Dwell In. If you turn away your foot from the Sabbath, from doing your pleasure on My holy day, and call the Sabbath a delight, the holy day of the* LORD *honorable, and shall honor Him, not doing your own ways, nor finding your own pleasure, nor speaking your own words, then you shall delight yourself in the* LORD*; and I will cause you to ride on the high hills of the earth, and feed you with the heritage of Jacob your father. The mouth of the* LORD *has spoken.*
>
> (Isaiah 58:5–14)

We should read these verses again and again. We should even commit them to memory to remind us of our duty toward others. In a world where the gulf between those who have and those who have not is ever widening, we need to be reminded to feed the hungry and clothe the poor; to help our own relatives, no matter how objectionable their lifestyle; to bring deliverance to the needy by breaking the bonds of wickedness as we bring them the light and truth of Jesus Christ; to give up vanity, fault-finding, and self-seeking. Yes, these are the verses that will remind us how to be more like Christ.

In the midst of these great humanitarian reminders and their promises of the light of Christ in our lives—our health springing forth speedily, and righteousness and glory becoming the trademarks of our lives—let's not forget what brings this about. Taking God's chosen fast inspires us to serve humanity. Fasting unto the Lord unlocks the most profound Christlike desires within us.

Jesus Christ undertook a consecration fast for forty days in the wilderness. His public ministry after His fast mirrors the truths of Isaiah 58. Our worship, supplication, and fasting unto the Lord would likewise unleash in us profound desires and power to serve humanity. All we need do is fast in consecration, honoring God by *"not doing your own ways, nor finding your own pleasure, nor speaking your own words"* (Isaiah 58:13).

When Elmer and I were missionaries in the Canal Zone, we visited the Calvary Assembly in Orlando, pastored by our good friends Roy and Pauline Harthern. At that time, Pauline was concluding a two-week fast and decided to give me an offering to buy a new dress. "You really shouldn't," I argued.

When she couldn't convince me, she finally opened her purse, and the dollars began to spill out. She said, "Look at all the grocery money I've been saving while fasting. You need a pretty new dress, and God has enabled me to supply it." I graciously accepted her kind gift. That's the kind of selfless giving that fasting should promote in our lives.

Opening Our Hearts to the Hungry

The experience of fasting, although not actual starvation, allows us to identify with those who must go without food unwillingly. The simulated starvation experience inherent in fasting opens our hearts to our needy neighbors. We realize what it feels like to be weak and in need of the strength food provides. We face the fear (simulated though it may be) of starvation. Through fasting, we can more fully sympathize with those for whom it is not a choice to go without food, but is in fact a terrifying way of life.

Years ago we pastored a church in Livermore, California. The six-member George Perkins family set aside one day every week to have a meal of only rice. Denying themselves the great abundance and variety of foods that Americans enjoy, they joined countless third-world families that subsist on such a simple meal. They gave to world missions the grocery money saved by partaking in this inexpensive meal. Surely we can think of similar ways to serve our brothers and sisters. Through prayer and fasting, as the verses in Isaiah promise, we don't even have to think of ways. The Lord will take care of that for us, in His own ways, in His own time.

Finally, St. Peter Chrysologus commented on the beauty of God's chosen fast when he said, "Fasting is the soul of prayer, and helping the needy is the lifeblood of fasting."

Interceding for Others

Have you ever given yourself to intercessory prayer for the needs of others? Why not give yourself to intercessory prayer and fasting? When we set aside our own needs and fast for the spiritual healing and renewal of others, this is intercessory fasting. God is pleased with such a sacrifice.

Moses demonstrated intercessory fasting in his dealings with the Israelites. During that time, God gave him the Ten Commandments. When Moses started down the mountain, he realized the whole nation had turned to idolatry. At that moment, he decided to undertake an intercessory fast on behalf of the people. Let's read Moses' own account:

> *Then I took the two tablets and threw them out of my two hands and broke them before your eyes. And I fell down before the* Lord*, as at the first, forty days and forty nights; I neither ate bread nor drank water, because of all your sin which you committed in doing wickedly in the sight of the* Lord *to provoke Him to anger. For I was afraid of the anger and hot displeasure with which the* Lord *was angry with you. But the* Lord *listened to me at that time also. And the Lord was very angry with Aaron and would have destroyed him; so I prayed for Aaron also at the same time."* (Deuteronomy 9:17–20)

Moses was the classic corporate personality who thought and acted in behalf of a body of people. The corporate personality is also seen when one person—a prophet, priest, or king—represents a body of people in a given cause. Moses did just this when he took upon himself the burden of the nation's sin through intercessory prayer and fasting.

Another example of a corporate personality is Ezekiel, who lay on his side for forty days to bear the punishment of the house of Judah. God told him, *"I have laid on you a day for each year"* (Ezekiel 4:5–6).

We can likewise invest ourselves in a consecrated fast for the sake of others. In effect, we stand in for them. We repent for the sins of our country, our friends, and our family. Of course, none of us can accept the Lord's forgiveness for others. They must do that for themselves. But we can intercede on their behalf, fasting and praying that they'll open themselves to God's forgiving love.

Jesus gave us an example when He interceded for others as He hung from the cross. In pure love, He said, *"Father, forgive them, for they do not know what they do"* (Luke 23:34). As I think of Jesus' example, I often remember my mother as she knelt in prayer. From the time I was able to walk, I can recall her kneeling beside her bed while tears streamed down her face. I touched the wet tears on her cheeks with my tiny hand. She put her arm around me, drew me close, and whispered in my ear, "Mommy is okay. She is just praying for the people who don't know Jesus."

After Jesus taught about the proper way to give, pray, and fast, He told His disciples, *"Lay up for yourselves treasures in heaven, where neither moth nor rust destroys and where thieves do not break in and steal"* (Matthew 6:20). By interceding, Mother called it "laying lambs at the feet of our Good Shepherd, Jesus." The lambs are our treasures. Jesus said, *"For where your treasure is, there your heart will be also"* (Matthew 6:21).

God Himself declared the power of intercessory prayer and fasting.

> *If My people who are called by My name will humble themselves, and pray and seek My face, and turn from their wicked ways, then will I hear from heaven, and will forgive their sin and heal their land. Now My eyes will be open and My ears attentive to prayer made in this place.*
>
> (2 Chronicles 7:14–15)

Developing Discipline

Fasting, a rigorous means to develop self-discipline, also measures the depth of our commitment to God. To undertake a fast means to be still while we allow the Spirit of God to lead us. While fasting, we wage war against the lust of the flesh, selfishness, rebellion, pride, and Satan's other weaponry cast for our personal destruction. While we fast unto the Lord, we also wage war with Satan. Our spiritual nature and our carnal existence come face-to-face in combat.

We have the potential to become spiritually strong enough to overcome any temptations that would sever us from our heavenly Father. When the perverted appetite and the inevitable seductions of food come while fasting, we must look to the Lord and rely on His strength. In fasting, we discipline ourselves to trust God. We learn that He will take care of us in our greatest moments of need, but in His time and in His way.

This final lesson to be learned while fasting unto the Lord is also the greatest lesson. As we discover the true and personal meaning of obedience and self-discipline through fasting, we come to appreciate the fullness of God. The simple Scripture so often quoted and so seldom pondered takes on newfound power: *"Man shall not live by bread alone"* (Matthew 4:4).

In light of these nine good reasons for undertaking a spiritual fast, the question shouldn't be, "Why fast unto the Lord?" Instead, we should ask ourselves, "Why not fast unto the Lord?"

Thirteen

When You Fast

"We're commanded to pray. We're commanded to give," a man once challenged me. "But show me just one New Testament command to fast." He consented that God's people often fasted in the early church. But this modern-day Christian argued, "God never *commanded* them to do it!"

I understand his reasoning. Until I was open to fasting, I found all kinds of ways to rationalize it out of my thoughts. Fasting meant going without food, and I didn't want to miss any meals. Fasting wasn't a popular topic, and I didn't want myself branded as being different or odd.

Fasting unto the Lord did not become a significant part of my life until God led me to a greater surrender to Jesus Christ. This doesn't mean I'm more spiritual than those who don't fast. I can only say that fasting was the next step—and a necessary one—in my own growth as a Christian.

If we can accept praying and giving as forms of worship practiced by God's people today, why not fasting? Scripture reveals that fasting unto the Lord assumes a place equal in importance to these two practices. Jesus' Sermon on the Mount presents the most direct lessons in giving, praying, and fasting that we can find in the Bible. Jesus warned against giving, praying, and fasting as purely external acts that bring self-glory, that make us *"like the hypocrites* [Pharisees]" (Matthew 6:16). Rather, these verses bring corrective instruction that teaches us to glorify God in our daily lives.

When You Give

In His Sermon on the Mount, Jesus contrasted how to give and how not to give. His teaching countered the false piety of the religious leaders of that day. His lesson on giving applies to us as much as it applied to those who heard Him preach it the first time:

> *Take heed that you do not do your charitable deeds before men, to be seen by them. Otherwise you have no reward from your Father in heaven. Therefore, when you do a charitable deed, do not sound a trumpet before you as the hypocrites do in the synagogues and in the streets, that they may have glory from men. Assuredly, I say to you, they have their reward. But when you do a charitable deed, do not let your left hand know what your right hand is doing, that your charitable deed may be in secret; and your Father who sees in secret will Himself reward you openly.*
>
> (Matthew 6:1–4)

Jesus taught His disciples to give in secret. We are not to boast to the world about what or how much we give. We shouldn't give to receive approval or commendation from others. God rewards our giving if we don't give out of prideful desire for personal recognition. Rather, we should give to please our heavenly Father. Jesus promises that God will reward us openly for doing this.

"In secret" does not mean that no one must know of the gift; it means that we should give quietly, humbly, without fanfare, and without seeking applause from others. Jesus couldn't have meant that all giving must be done without anyone knowing. If that were true, we could never write a check to the church or make a pledge for the building fund.

When You Pray

Christ lived a life of prayer, seeking the fellowship of His heavenly Father long before the activity of the day began. He often withdrew from the crowds to gain new strength and direction in God's presence. In addition to modeling a life of prayer, Christ also taught us how to pray and how not to pray:

> *And when you pray, you shall not be like the hypocrites. For they love to pray standing in the synagogues and on the comers of the streets, that they may be seen by men. Assuredly, I say to you, they have their reward. But you, when you pray, go into your room, and when you have shut your door, pray to your Father who is in the secret place; and your Father who sees in secret will reward you openly. And when you pray, do not use vain repetitions as the heathen do. For they think that they will be heard for their many words. Therefore do not be like them. For your*

> *Father knows the things you have need of before you ask Him.* (Matthew 6:5–8)

God's lessons are clear. We should pray privately—in our hearts, that is, in our "closets." Jesus didn't mean that we should never pray in public. If that were the case, we couldn't come together and pray in church as the body of Christ. Although we may pray in a group, it should be a secret, personal, heartfelt prayer. We are not to pray in such a way that we put on a show. We are not ever to pray to impress others with prideful self-righteousness.

As with giving correctly, Jesus promises us that if we pray with clean hearts, God will reward us openly. The most obvious reward is, of course, the answered prayer. When Christians pray with the right motives, according to Christ's instructions, they will receive a spiritual reward.

When You Fast

In His Sermon on the Mount, Jesus Christ taught the lesson that is the primary subject of this book—how not to fast unto the Lord and how to fast unto the Lord:

> *Moreover, when you fast, do not be like the hypocrites, with a sad countenance. For they disfigure their faces that they may appear to men to be fasting. Assuredly, I say to you, they have their reward. But you, when you fast, anoint your head and wash your face, so that you do not appear to men to be fasting, but to your Father who is in the secret place; and your Father who sees in secret will reward you openly.*
> (Matthew 6:16–18)

Like His lessons on giving and praying, Jesus' instructions on fasting are perfectly clear. We are to fast in a right spirit. We are not to walk around with a solemn face as we cast ourselves as self-sacrificing sufferers. Jesus Christ specifically instructs us not to fast in pretense, *"like the hypocrites, with a sad countenance,"* who attempt to win the sympathy of others. Nor are we to fast in order to be held in awe or to gain the admiration through a counterfeit spirit of self-righteous piety. We should never fast in the spirit of a melodramatic actor seeking an audience's praise. We need to consider fasting, like any other form of self-discipline, as a means to glorify God as we grow in grace. If we lose sight of this pursuit, fasting becomes mere ritual, a selfish move to earn God's grace, or an empty act of false piety.

Undertaking a fast should be a mature response to the Holy Spirit speaking to us. Fasting is a pure message to ourselves and to God that we treasure *"the words of His mouth more than* [our] *necessary food"* (Job 23:12). We should fast in the same spirit as we are to give and to pray—humbly and with a right heart. (We do not have to keep fasting an absolute secret: we simply have to fast with a right heart.) And when we fast—as when we give and pray—Jesus promises that God will reward us openly.

Just as all praying is not done in a secret chamber and all giving is not done in secret, neither is all fasting expected to be completely undisclosed. Christ gave His disciples the same message for giving, praying, and fasting. We should not announce the spiritual fast by purposefully looking peaked, gray, or sick in order to draw sympathy from the world. Trying to impress others with our supposed spirituality reveals misguided motivation. If fasting is done in this way, Jesus warned that the applause and sympathy we receive would be our only reward. Fasters would completely miss the spiritual benefits of our heavenly Father's reward.

Why do we understand Christ's teachings on giving and praying but misinterpret His instructions on fasting? The answer is twofold. First, living in our affluent culture, it's easier to give money from our wallets than to withhold food from our mouths. It's also easier to spend a few minutes in prayer than it is to deny our appetites and pleasures. Second, most of us receive no instructions or encouragement to fast. If anything, we receive put-downs, fear tactics, or indifference when we bring up the topic. Peer pressure and taking the easy way to God win over fasting nearly every time.

Some of us make fasting unattractive. We try to follow Jesus' instructions too rigidly. We may unintentionally misinterpret, putting more importance on keeping the fast a secret rather than on the emphasis of worship and fellowship with God. With this misinterpretation of Scripture, it is no wonder that fasting has become difficult. How often can anyone do anything for any length of time, especially involving days or weeks, completely in secret? Could this also be one more reason why we neglect fasting?

In one of our seminars on fasting held in Albuquerque, a man shared with us, "My wife doesn't like it when I fast. She really gets angry when I don't eat with her." He later revealed he never told her he was fasting until the meal was ready. He was trying to keep his fasting "a secret." What woman would appreciate such a surprise? A man should let his wife know ahead of time that he will be forgoing her culinary treats for the day by simply saying, "I am fasting today, so I won't be eating tonight." This is not only common courtesy; it is also common sense!

Some people try to be so secretive about fasting that they draw attention to themselves, causing others to wonder what could possibly be wrong with them. These secret fasters sit in the restaurant with their friends and when someone wonders why they are just drinking water, they won't say. Finally, someone catches on and whispers to the others, "I think Bill is fasting." It eliminates the secrecy and awkwardness of such situations if those choosing to fast just explain, "Please excuse me for not ordering, but I am fasting today."

If the faster cares to share the reason for his fast, his explanation might even be an opportunity for his friends to agree with him in prayer. If not, no long dissertation on the virtues of fasting is necessary. The explanation is enough. He has broken no scriptural rule.

Similar Disciplines

In Matthew 6, Christ undoubtedly assumed that as Christians and lovers of God we would automatically give, pray, and fast. His primary concern was to teach us how and how not to practice these disciplines. All three of these forms of worship—giving, praying, and fasting—are intertwined in time and spirit throughout the Sermon on the Mount. Notice, for instance, the parallel construction of each of the three messages:

1. Jesus warned His disciples how not to give, pray, and fast.

2. He warned them that a worldly reward is all they will receive if they refuse to be forewarned.
3. He taught them how to give, pray, and fast.
4. He assured them that following His instructions would result in God rewarding them openly.

Jesus intentionally used identical parallel construction in these verses to teach all Christians that these three disciplines—giving, praying, and fasting—should take parallel importance in their lives. Note His choice of words in the following verses:

When you do a charitable deed.... (Matthew 6:2)

When you pray.... (Matthew 6:5)

Moreover, when you fast.... (Matthew 6:16)

The key words are the temporal indicators, identical in each verse: *when.* Notice that Jesus didn't say "if" in His teachings. Jesus assumed that His listeners practiced all three disciplines. He wanted to present corrective teaching on how to do each in the proper spirit. We can infer from this passage that Jesus interwove giving, praying, and fasting together, one as essential as the next, in creating the strong fabric of the full Christian life.

Why has the church recognized giving and praying as elements of Christian commitment to the Lord, while we ignore or dispute fasting? A study of Scripture easily proves that we have as much if not more proof in support of fasting as we do for giving, and nearly as much as for praying. Because of this, isn't it strange that we understand Christ's exhortations on giving and prayer, but our attention fades when we read His principles of fasting?

Why Do We Neglect Fasting?

Today, we can still profit from the teachings of Jesus Christ in His Sermon on the Mount. But we also need basic information about fasting. We still pray; we still give; but we shrink back from fasting. Why is this so? Why has fasting been relegated to a practice of the early church and is hardly a common occurrence today? Besides all the other reasons that explain why we leave fasting out of our lives today, the following three reasons deserve consideration:

1. *We neglect fasting because we fear self-abuse.* Isolated, rare cases of horrifying abuse of fasting leave us feeling that fasting is better left to the ancients. In the early 1980s, I heard that a devout man in Chicago died while on his knees—on the sixtieth day of his fast. Such abuse of fasting brings no glory to God. Lengthy fasts, especially in a depleted state of ill health, need supervision to avoid such tragedies.

Fasting fell into abuse during the Middle Ages. Remember, fasting has a long history. The Pharisees practiced fasting as a badge of spiritual pride. During the Dark Ages, this practice regained popularity. Emaciated cheeks and skeletal frames were the marks of the most spiritual among men. As true spirituality declined, church people turned to any ritual that would give them the veneer of true spirituality. The practice of fasting was a favorite, especially among the monks. Fasting as a form of worship became divested of its spiritual power. Formalities and ritual took over.

As a discipline, fasting came under the most rigid regulations during these dark times. Monks particularly practiced self-flagellation and self-mortification in their attempt at purifying themselves through fasting. This was an abuse of fasting. Although we may have never studied these historical times for ourselves, the folklore of fasting as abuse has become a part of us. This folklore makes one perfectly good reason to neglect the practice in our daily lives.

2. *We neglect fasting because of deception.* Included in this reason for leaving fasting to the ancients are all the rationalizations presented in this book. Deception is just another word for rationalization.

The commercial food giants and mass media have collaborated to flood us with messages to eat. We are overwhelmed with propaganda telling us that we must eat three large meals a day, with plenty of snacks and coffee breaks in between. We are deceived into thinking that if we miss one meal, we are teetering on the precipice of starvation.

But we are not deceived by the food giants and profit makers alone. Deception comes from within, too. Self-deception comes in the form of our parroting all the folklore, myths, and miseducation we have ever heard:

"Doesn't fasting destroy healthy body tissue?"

"If I fast, I get so weak that I can't work. How many of us can take time off from work for that?"

"I've heard that you can injure your health permanently by fasting—it can even kill you!"

"I tried fasting twice and quit. I couldn't do anything but think about food. So I figured I might as well eat if I was going to go crazy thinking about food!"

From what we have learned about fasting so far, these statements sound ridiculous. Because our minds are constantly thinking about food, that's all the more reason we need to fast—so that food does not control our thinking and our bellies do not become our gods.

The most shocking statement of self-delusion I ever heard came from a well-known Christian singer. She weighed over 300 pounds when she seriously explained why she had neglected fasting to enrich her spiritual life: "I have heard that fasting destroys the brain cells."

As mentioned in an earlier chapter, experienced scientists and doctors who have supervised hundreds of thousands of fasts in this century can verify the fallacy of this woman's thinking. When we fast, the body lives on its reserves, its nonessential tissues, and its waste and morbid tissue.

3. *We neglect fasting out of ignorance.* When nobody knows anything about it, nobody does it. Everybody says fasting is for the olden days, so why should the twenty-first century Christian be motivated to fast?

I have been in the church all my life. I never heard much about fasting—at least not for today. I read about it in the Bible, of course. When I examined the writings of the great saints, I discovered that most of them fasted. But like most believers, I never learned to apply fasting to my own life. I simply lived in ignorance.

Yes, ignorance on the practice of fasting abounds among even the more seasoned Christian leaders. A seminary student proved this when he published the results of research required for his graduate theology degree. He sent a questionnaire to over three hundred church leaders. His final question asked, "Do you think that fasting would develop your Christian life?"

The answers went like this:

- 55 replied, "Yes." (A few qualified their answers with statements such as "if done correctly" or "only if led by the Holy Spirit.")
- 32 replied, "No." (One responded, "No! No! No!")
- 83 replied, "Perhaps," "Possibly," "Not sure," or "Need to think more about it."

While this survey has no statistical significance because of its small sampling, the results indicate how little God's people know about fasting. Worse yet, our church leaders have been willing to skip right over the fasting section of the most famous sermon ever given.

The only way to dispel the darkness of abuse, deception, and ignorance about fasting is to step into the full light of Jesus Christ. The Sermon on the Mount is all the truth we need to convince us of the importance of fasting. Fasting is parallel to both giving and praying. Without a doubt, fasting should be every bit as much a part of our spiritual lives as tithing and prayerful worship.

We can find other areas of the Bible that further dispel the darkness that surrounds fasting. Consider the specific command to fast in the Old Testament that revolves around the Day of Atonement. In addition, the Jews had other times of fasting. Queen Esther instituted an annual fast called the Fast of Purim. The prophets often proclaimed fasts for specific purposes and of limited duration as they called the people to humble themselves before God.

A few examples of fasters include Moses, Hannah, Samuel, David, Elijah, Esther, Daniel, Ezra, Nehemiah,

Anna the prophetess, and the apostle Paul. Do you still doubt that fasting was a well-used route to know the heart of God? Here are some well-known people who fasted:

- Hannah, after being taunted, fasted and prayed for God to give her a child. (See 1 Samuel 1:1–7.)
- Samuel led the nation in fasting for their sinful ways at Mizpah. (See 1 Samuel 7:5–6.)
- David fasted when his son by Bathsheba was dying. (See 2 Samuel 12:15–16.)
- Daniel fasted when he sought special guidance from God. (See Daniel 10:1–12.)
- Esther fasted before making her request to King Ahasuerus. (See Esther 4:15–16.)
- Paul and Barnabas fasted before they appointed elders. (See Acts 14:23.)
- Church leaders at Antioch fasted before sending Paul and Barnabas as their first missionaries. (See Acts 13:1–3.)

Some great leaders of the Christian church were great advocates of fasting: St. Teresa of Avila, Martin Luther, Joan of Arc, John Calvin, John Knox, John Wesley, John Bunyan, Jonathan Edwards, David Brainerd, and Charles Finney. All these people believed in fasting and held it in high regard. That doesn't make it mandatory. But those of us who seek more of God in our lives may want to add fasting to our giving and praying in order to seek Him more fully.

People often speak of their desire to walk more closely with God. I don't question their desire. But if we want that precious intimacy with God, we need to avail ourselves of all the means that God offers us. The Sermon on the Mount explains the three most powerful means to find that closeness: we must give, we must pray, and we must fast.

Fourteen

How to Fast unto the Lord

For months the funds for our television ministry continued to dwindle. Because of our commitment to reach the Spanish-speaking world, Elmer and I could not understand why our resources were at low ebb. We prayed. We worked hard. Yet even Elmer's constant travel to raise funds barely kept Buenos Amigos on the air.

We used every dime from our fund-raising to cover office expenses and our employee payroll. We could barely pay our part-time secretary and our son, Chris, who produced our TV programs. Both of them were already working for us at a personal sacrifice. They sometimes had to wait for weeks to cash their payroll checks. I was embarrassed to ask them to wait. In the midst of what felt like failure, I strongly talked of trusting God—and we did. Yet we saw no visible signs of improvement.

We took care of our personal needs only after we paid our ministry bills. Too often we barely managed to pay our ministry expenses with nothing left over. The pressure of creditors wanting their money drove me to utter helplessness and frustration. Production money being virtually nonexistent, we couldn't take advantage of any opportunity to add any new programs. Our old ones had run their course, and few stations wanted to continue playing them.

"If God wants us to continue in this part of our ministry, then He will provide the money," I told my husband firmly. "Furthermore, if we don't have the money to support our ministry, I don't feel it's right to use our rent money to pay for it." I didn't mind making personal sacrifices when I knew God was leading us. Yet I also believed that God cares for His own. As Christians and good stewards, we should have enough money to pay our bills and to provide for our needs.

I wasn't questioning God so much as I was confused on where we were failing. My heavy heart urged me to get alone and open myself to God without interruption. I chose an isolated spot in Death Valley to spend eight days alone with God. My morning walks started my day in communion with Him. I determined, through prayer and fasting, to find the way back to order, peace, and joyful prosperity in our lives.

I arose before dawn and went out for what would become the first of eight desert walks. I had been here many times before and looked forward to the breathtaking desert sunrises each day. The beauty of Death Valley always had a calming effect on me, and I always felt close to God here.

On that first morning walk, I started to pray. I soon felt an agonizing heaviness inside. My tongue seemed to be stuck to the roof of my mouth. I clutched my chest. The emotional pain threatened to take all the breath out of my body.

Memories of sermons telling me to be specific in prayer rang in my ears. I drew another deep breath to drive out the crushing pain in my chest. I whispered, "God, how can I be specific when I don't even know how or what to pray for? If I had the answer, I wouldn't have the problem!" I could only point to my dilemma and plead, "God, look at the mess we're in. How do I pray? How can I pray?"

Later I went back into my rustic cabin and sat on the bed. Opening my Bible to Romans, I glanced down, hardly knowing where to begin. I read page after page, but nothing penetrated my consciousness until I got to the eighth chapter:

> *For we do not know what we should pray for as we ought, but the Spirit Himself makes intercession for us with groanings which cannot be uttered. Now He who searches the hearts knows what the mind of the Spirit is, because He makes intercession for the saints according to the will of God.* (Romans 8:26–27)

Upon reading that passage, a great sense of relief came over me. I didn't worry about being specific any longer. I was confident that the Holy Spirit knew not only my needs, but also how to best lead me to the answers. After starting to pray, I sensed God's Spirit praying through me.

I prayed in a new kind of way, with a groaning that started from the deepest part of me. Feeling the Spirit of God praying through my body, I poured myself out in intense intercession. My heaviness changed to great sorrow. I was deep in mourning. Contrition for failure and anguish for weakness struggled inside me.

Wordlessly I groaned, as if waiting for new strength to come so that I could go back into the spiritual foray once again.

The next morning, I became acutely aware that Satan had opposed us. I sensed his power and determination to win over me and over our family ministry. This was a battle I had to win. Boldness replaced the crushing pain in my chest, and I vented my anger on him. Alone on the desert, I rejoiced as I raised my voice to rebuke Satan.

I fought to regain from Satan the freedom that rightfully belonged to us. I fought to restore peace in our home that now suffered from Satan's worldly pressures. I fought for the release of Satan's stronghold on our television ministry. I fought for order, peace, and joyful prosperity for our lives in the name of Jesus.

This spiritual battle and prayerful war paralleled the truth of the following verse:

> *We do not wrestle against flesh and blood, but against principalities, against powers, against the rulers of the darkness of this age, against spiritual hosts of wickedness in the heavenly places.* (Ephesians 6:12)

Among the cacti and sand, I realized that Jesus defeated Satan in a desert similar to this, which energized me even more. When my prayer battle ended, I knew that I, too, had triumphed over Satan. I picked up the spoils of the victory—my freedom, my peace, and my joy—and returned to the cabin.

On the third morning, I carefully reviewed our ministry over the past twenty years. In the beginning,

God had called Elmer and me to carry out His vision. God had made it perfectly clear that we were to have this ministry, that we were to continue, and that it was to thrive. We simply needed to change the way we executed the ministry as we responded to God's call.

By the end of the week, I had claimed a victory over Satan. Without a doubt, I knew he was defeated. Drained from this spiritual warfare, I wanted to stay on awhile, resting in the Lord's good graces. I wasn't quite ready to leave my hideaway, but my schedule wouldn't let me stay any longer.

The time was not right to share my triumphant prayer battle with anyone, so I kept silent upon my return. I decided to wait, praising God for our victory, even though the outward circumstances had not changed in my absence.

On my first day back in the office, our son, Chris, greeted me with enthusiasm. "Mom! I've got an idea! Remember that Christmas special we made a few years ago? The music is still up-to-date, and it even has an excellent dramatization. It never got a lot of air time, so few people have seen it. It's still on the shelf in our video storage room. Why don't we duplicate it and offer it to the stations that used to air our programs? Maybe they'll air it this Christmas season, free of charge."

Knowing that air time is not free—not even on Christian radio and television—and that the secular stations where we usually air our programs charge even more, I hesitated and then uttered, "All right."

"Wait a minute!" Chris interrupted as his eyes brightened with excitement. "Why not ask the stations if they will *buy* the program?"

A revolutionary approach. We didn't know anyone who had ever sold a Christian program to secular stations. Nevertheless, Elmer and I encouraged him to go ahead.

Chris got on the phone, duplicated tapes, made all the arrangements, and sent the program by special courier to the stations in time for Christmas. And the idea worked! A few months later, we followed with an Easter program. The stations either aired it free or paid for the privilege of running it. Over two hundred secular TV stations with nationwide coverage in fifteen Latin countries broadcast the show. In one country we even replaced the evening news on Christmas Eve!

Our priorities were adjusted, finances improved, and soon we were in control—all with the help of almighty God. I'm not so presumptuous to think it happened because of my prayers alone. Elmer, Chris, and our daughter, Kim, fasted and prayed as well.

Why hadn't we thought of this plan before? I believe we had to battle it out with prayer and fasting. My part was to claim a victory over our adversary during my prayer time in the desert. God set us free. The fasting and intercession had helped to release God's creative power in Chris.

My mourning was turned into joy, just as Isaiah 61:3 promises. This dramatic answer to fasting, coupled with reflections on my own experiences, stirred my longing to discover more about this neglected discipline. I started studying the passages that taught us the proper way to fast unto the Lord.

Wine and Wineskins

First, I studied the concept of old wine and old wineskins, as compared with new wine and new wineskins. This metaphor opened the way to understand the new order of New Testament fasting. Jesus explained the metaphor as follows:

> *No one puts a piece of unshrunk cloth on an old garment; for the patch pulls away from the garment, and the tear is made worse. Nor do they put new wine into old wineskins, or else the wineskins break, the wine is spilled, and the wineskins are ruined. But they put new wine into new wineskins, and both are preserved.*
>
> (Matthew 9:16–17)

Jesus taught us how to cultivate a deeper relationship with God. We have a responsibility to live godly, purposeful lives. By instruction and through example, Jesus unfolded the divine plan in its fullness to help us carry out God's will.

The Old Testament law is the written will of God given to a particular nation for a particular period of time—until the coming of God's Son. The Mosaic law is unchangeable and continues as a prophetic preparation for the second coming of Christ. The Mosaic law also paved the way for the first coming of Christ.

Jesus presented the New Testament practices of giving, praying, and fasting, which replaced the old and which are still fully valid today. In the Sermon on the Mount, Jesus warned us against turning these practices into mere ritual and false piety. God wants us to give, pray, and fast with only the purest motives, exclusively for Him who sees in secret.

The new and greater law of righteousness that Jesus brought, however, places us on an honor system. Rules, regulations, and formalities are not to burden us any longer. Now we must allow the Holy Spirit to lead us in fulfilling God's will. Jesus Christ showed us how to be motivated by love in all we do.

Jesus gave new instruction on fasting that abolished the Old Testament customs and traditions—the old wineskins. By using the metaphor of the new wineskins and the old, His hearers saw that the old customs were the old wineskins. They also understood that Christ brought new wine to fill His followers. Therefore, He had to prepare the new wineskins—the new ways—for the preservation of both.

What about Mourning?

In many places throughout Scripture, the word *mourning* can be used interchangeably with *fasting*. For instance, when Daniel referred to his twenty-one day fast, he said, *"In those days I, Daniel, was **mourning** three full weeks"* (Daniel 10:2, emphasis added).

The New Testament also supports this truth. When the disciples of John the Baptist asked why they fasted and Jesus' disciples didn't, Jesus replied,

> *Can the friends of the bridegroom **mourn** as long as the bridegroom is with them? But the days will come when the bridegroom will be taken away from them, and then they will fast.*
>
> (Matthew 9:15, emphasis added)

Jesus used the word *mourn* to indicate that while He was with His disciples—while the bridegroom was present—it wasn't the proper time to fast.

During that historical period, fasting usually marked a critical time or a time of mourning. Jesus' life on earth marked a time of joyous celebration! Why would the disciples want to mourn when the Bridegroom was with them? No one could be sad in His presence! If the wedding guests cannot mourn, it would be impossible for them to fast because the two invariably went together. Historically, therefore, this period of feasting and celebration shared by Jesus' disciples in His presence was an exception.

Jesus emphasized the spirit of the final age beginning with Him. For this reason, His disciples were not known for their fasting. Although the new age began with Him, fasting would continue as a sign of worship on this earth. He also said that His disciples would mourn after the Bridegroom was taken away, but because of the expectation of His second coming, fasting would be practiced with new meaning. Mourning would be intermixed with joy. (See Isaiah 61:3.)

Fasting would be a sad memorial of what happened on that Passover weekend, but it would also be intermixed with inner confidence and simple trust in His second coming. The New Testament fast, therefore, was something new and distinct from previous practices. The Christian basis for fasting—the sacrifice of Jesus—and the inner confidence, trust, and joy motivated by His love make fasting an entirely different experience than the traditional Judaic fast. God has set His children free from sin. With that freedom, we also enjoy our glorious salvation, which gives us a new and stronger basis for fasting unto the Lord.

Matthew used *mourning* rather than *fasting* because it characterized how Christians wait for the second coming of Christ. We can infer from the Beatitudes that the word *mourn* can include fasting and probably did in the early church. *"Blessed are those who mourn* [that probably includes "those who fast"], *for they shall be comforted"* (Matthew 5:4). In commenting on Matthew 5:4, one author wrote,

> His gift of happiness is for those who mourn for themselves. They sense their failures and want to do something about them. They grieve because they have not fully lived up to their understanding of God's claims on their lives.[1]

While the biblical writers did not always use a particular word or phrase such as *mourning* or *fasting* to record times when people fasted unto the Lord, there are, nevertheless, many instances of lamentation or deep sadness where the ancients undoubtedly fasted.

1. For defeat in battle. (See Judges 20:25–26.)
2. For sad tidings. (See Nehemiah 1:4.)
3. For a plague. (See Joel 1:2–4, 13–14; 2:12–15.)
4. For the threat of disaster. (See 2 Chronicles 20:1–3; Esther 4:3; 9:30–31.)

Don't Wear Sackcloth and Ashes

Jesus carefully instructed His disciples by referring to the shortcomings of the Pharisees. *"Moreover, when you fast, do not be like the hypocrites, with a sad countenance. For they disfigure their faces that they may appear to men to be fasting"* (Matthew 6:16). Jesus admonished His followers that fasting for pretended piety exposed wrong motives. Fasting would then become nothing more than an exercise to show the world how devoted and self-disciplined one was, rather than a form of true worship. Jesus condemned this fasting when it was an ostentatious parade of prideful piety.

Jesus knew the Pharisees had purposely chosen Monday and Thursday to fast because those days coincided with market days. People from the countryside crowded the villages, and many flocked to Jerusalem. Those who fasted for show had a greater audience on these days. The Pharisees walked through the streets dressed in a scratchy burlap called sackcloth and powdered their faces with ashes as signs of their sacrifice.

Wearing sackcloth had originally symbolized a *"spirit of heaviness"* (Isaiah 61:3). Isaiah said that this *"spirit of heaviness"* would be changed to a *"garment of praise"* (verse 3). Isaiah prophesied that this mourning apparel would eventually express praise and gratitude instead of a spirit of heaviness.

This mourning, or spirit of heaviness, had been the Old Testament mood of fasting: the people felt a heavy burden for their own needs and for the needs of others. New Testament fasting would still have that seriousness, but it would also bring praise, joy, and gratitude to the faster. Whenever Jesus was moved with compassion while He was on earth, He responded positively to the situation. This same compassion moves sensitive believers who have burdened spirits to respond in intercessory prayer and fasting.

Besides donning sackcloth, the Pharisees whitened their faces with ashes to accentuate their paleness.

During a fast they didn't bathe or wash any part of their bodies. Men didn't trim their beards. This helped them create the look of sacrifice and sadness they imagined holy fasters to wear.

Fasting, which had begun as an act of genuine contrition and deep sorrow for sin, eventually became a ritual. The uncomfortable sackcloth symbolized self-sacrifice, and the ashes symbolized suffering. Both were designed to evoke the admiration of the passersby and then to elicit their great sympathy.[2] How did Jesus respond to such a pretentious, outward show of what should have been a secret, inner discipline? He told His disciples, *"Assuredly, I say to you, they have their reward"* (Matthew 6:16).

Anoint with Oil

Jesus rebuked the false piety of the Pharisees, but He also instructed His disciples how to fast. *"But you, when you fast, anoint your head and wash your face"* (Matthew 6:17). These instructions were opposed to the common practice of His day. The Pharisees strictly forbade washing the face and anointing the head during a fast.

Like the Pharisees, the ancients didn't use oil during a fast. Since oil represented joy, it was commonly used to anoint kings, priests, and prophets. Anointing with oil was a common practice during times of festivity and gladness but never during times of grief and mourning. Jewish law forbid the use of oil while fasting or mourning. Consider these examples of Old Testament anointing:

• During Daniel's fast, he said, *"I, Daniel, was mourning three full weeks. I ate no pleasant food, no*

meat or wine came into my mouth, nor did I anoint myself at all, till three whole weeks were fulfilled" (Daniel 10:2–3).

• Joab plotted to reconcile David to Absalom. He hired a wise woman who pretended to be in mourning. He instructed her, *"Put on mourning apparel* [sackcloth]*; do not anoint yourself with oil"* (2 Samuel 14:2).

• When David broke his fast, he anointed himself, signaling he had stopped. *"So David arose from the ground, washed and anointed himself, and changed his clothes; and he went into the house of the LORD and worshiped. Then he went to his own house; and when he requested, they set food before him, and he ate"* (2 Samuel 12:20).

• Isaiah prophesied that Christ was going to give *"the oil of joy for mourning"* (Isaiah 61:3). Jesus' instruction to anoint the head with oil during a fast represented the new wineskins designed to hold new wine.

Jesus changed the anointing customs once and for all. Washing the face and anointing the head with oil became the new way to fast. Christ's disciples didn't need to smear ashes on their faces. Jesus told them to wash their faces. (See Matthew 6:17.) Isaiah prophesied this exchange: *"To console those who mourn in Zion, to give them beauty for ashes"* (Isaiah 61:3).

Undergo Affliction

Fasting is also associated with affliction. Ezra announced, *"Then I proclaimed a fast there, at the river Ahava, that we might afflict ourselves before our God"*

(Ezra 8:21 KJV). Leviticus records the only fast God Himself called in the Bible: *"And this shall be a statute for ever unto you: that in the seventh month, on the tenth day of the month, ye shall afflict your souls"* (Leviticus 16:29 KJV).

To "afflict our souls" shows our contempt for our wrongful deeds. God had the Israelites commemorate the most important day for affliction on their calendar with a fast. He could have chosen a feast, but He didn't. This shows the value God placed on the practice of fasting.

Scripture says, *"Humble yourselves in the sight of the Lord, and He will lift you up"* (James 4:10). In the Bible, people humbled themselves by fasting. God promises that such humbling will be well rewarded:

> *If My people who are called by My name will humble themselves, and pray and seek My face, and turn from their wicked ways, then I will hear from heaven, and will forgive their sin and heal their land. Now My eyes will be open and My ear attentive to prayer made in this place.*
>
> (2 Chronicles 7:14–15)

David mentioned the practice of fasting unto the Lord in his psalms: *"But as for me, when they were sick, my clothing was sackcloth; I humbled myself with fasting"* (Psalm 35:13). In another psalm he wrote, *"I wept and chastened my soul with fasting"* (Psalm 69:10).

Fasting provides the opportunity to show personal humility before God and to plead for mercy—not to force His hand. The king of Nineveh exhorted his people to fast, repent, and plead for mercy. He urged his citizens, *"Cry mightily to God....Who can tell if God will turn and relent, and turn away from His fierce anger, so that we may not perish?"* (Jonah 3:8–9).

But all this self-effacement does have its recompense. Nowhere is the rich reward of fasting unto the Lord made clearer than in Jesus' words, *"He who humbles himself win be exalted"* (Matthew 23:12).

Self-denial

Humility and self-denial are two sides of the same spiritual coin. In order to deny ourselves at our own expense and for the benefit of another, we must have humility in our hearts. Jesus' greatest calling to deny ourselves came when He stated, *"If anyone desires to come after Me, let him deny himself, and take up his cross, and follow Me"* (Matthew 16:24).

Built into this ultimate denial of "taking up the cross" is the denial inherent in fasting unto the Lord. Fasting denies that which legitimately belongs to us: the joy of eating. In fasting unto the Lord, we participate in Christ's redemptive suffering. By fasting unto the Lord, we answer His call to deny ourselves for the sake of the cross.

One day I asked myself, "Why is it so important to deny myself?" Immediately, I thought of a spoiled child who always gets his own way. No one can stand to be around selfish people who have no depth, no integrity, and no strength of character. Practicing self-denial builds character. Our personal acts of self-denial encourage us to seek the Lord more fully and to become more like Christ.

Scripture points out the value of self-denial: *"For if you live according to the flesh, you will die; but if by the Spirit you put to death the deeds of the body, you will live"* (Romans 8:13). God's call to deny ourselves assures us rewards.

"Give, and it will be given to you" (Luke 6:38). Jesus promised, *"He who finds his life will lose it, and he who loses his life for My sake will find it"* (Matthew 10:39). The way to glorify God and to become more like Christ is through the narrow road of self-denial. And what more demanding way to deny self than to fast unto the Lord?

Although I had heard about self-denial all my life, the reality of it did not dawn on me until the birth of our first child. Chris was five days old when we brought him home from the hospital. A few days later, Elmer decided to take me out for dinner at seven o'clock. About five in the afternoon, I began getting our new baby ready to go out with us. I bathed, dressed, and fed him. I prepared the formula, fined the bottles, folded the diapers, and packed the diaper bag.

Feeling a bit tired, I sat down on the bed to catch my breath. I glanced at the clock to find that it was already 7:00 P.M. It was time to leave, and I wasn't ready myself yet. That was a rude awakening. I said to myself, "Lee, it's never again going to be like it used to be. Your lifestyle has drastically changed. No longer will you have a lot of time for yourself." I dressed hurriedly, and we went to dinner a little late. In the years to follow, I quickly learned to readjust my schedule to accommodate Chris. I no longer had luxury time for myself. I was learning to deny myself for the sake of my son. Some of the privileges I had enjoyed and taken for granted were sacrificed out of love. I did not resent the sacrifice. I was happy to do it for the sake of love.

Motherhood has taught me one of the most precious lessons in life: the self-centered person can never find fulfillment or joy. Why? Because the Christian life is the continuing process of spiritual growth through self-denial. Selflessness is the way we find true fulfillment and joy.

Christ's love is not cheap. Christ does not offer salvation like some leftover carelessly discarded in the giveaway bin at a supermarket. Christ's love does not come easily. After all, nothing good comes free and easy! Salvation cost Christ His life! Wondrous privileges and weighty responsibilities accompany the gift of salvation.

The apostle Peter said,

> *Since Christ suffered and underwent pain, you must have the same attitude he did; you must be ready to suffer, too. For remember, when your body suffers, sin loses its power, and you won't be spending the rest of your life chasing after evil desires, but will be anxious to do the will of God.* (1 Peter 4:1–2 TLB)

The apostle Paul also expressed the beauty and costliness of Christ's love:

> *Now I have given up everything else—I have found it to be the only way to really know Christ and to experience the mighty power that brought him back to life again, and to find out what it means to suffer and to die with him.*
> (Philippians 3:10 TLB)

Paul recognized that Christ's sacrifice is far more than fair in its trade-off. *"For I consider that the sufferings of this present time are not worthy to be compared with the glory which shall be revealed in us"* (Romans 8:18).

Purified through Fasting

The sacrificial act of fasting unto the Lord leads to a better understanding of our relationship with ourselves, with others, with the world, and with God through Christ. Fasting burns out our selfishness. In fasting we willingly submit to the cauldron of renunciation as we give up one of life's greatest pleasures. Fasting is the foundry in which we are purified. Its fires refine our faith; its flames separate the base impurities from our true character in Christ; its hot blasts purify our hearts.

After fasting, we cool into tempered Christians, strong with self-control. The dross and cinders of our lustful cravings are skimmed off us during fasting. Fasting is the Lord's furnace over which our earthly slag is melted and removed so that the remaining pure gold may be cast into God's purpose. Today, fasting unto the Lord is nearly a lost art, yet we should not underestimate its value. Fasting produces a work of art—the tempered, selfless Christian—that can be created through no other process of refinement.

We can appreciate the burning desire of Christ's disciples to remove the human dross of temptation, cravings, and selfishness from their lives with fasting. We can understand why they chose to fast unto the Lord to expedite this process. Fasting and prayer powerfully bring temptations, cravings, and selfishness to the cross. We sacrifice the flesh for the sake of that final wedding feast when we will sup with the Bridegroom. We will find our love perfected and our souls purified by fasting unto the Lord. When our pilgrimage is enhanced with fasting unto the Lord, we add immeasurably to the fullness of our lives.

New Testament fasting and prayer take on new meaning and purpose. Jesus taught His disciples to pray, *"Your kingdom come. Your will be done on earth as it is in heaven"* (Matthew 6:10). Fasting and prayer help to bring the will of our heavenly Father to earth. God accomplishes His will for the world through His faithful intercessors.

The new instructions for fasting provided in the Sermon on the Mount were part of Christ's program for His new kingdom. Jesus lashed out at impious practices to ensure that His followers didn't emulate Judaizers or Pharisees who held onto old, dead rituals. The Christian fast was to be entirely new and decidedly different, especially in terms of inner motivation.

Jesus' concern was with the inner man. He asked His followers to fast with only the purest of motives. (See Matthew 6:17–18.) Because fasting requires the ultimate discipline, Christians need to understand God's true purpose. Once we accept and practice fasting as a Christian duty, rewards will surely follow. The power of food will be exchanged for the miracle-working power of the fast.

Fifteen

Questions on Fasting

When people come to our Genesis 1:29 seminars, they often have mixed feelings about fasting. Many of them have never fasted a day in their lives. Some have fasted for short durations but have never considered the longer consecration or therapeutic fasts. Others question whether fasting really yields both spiritual and physical benefits.

Most of our seminars include a lively question and answer session. Our informative dialogue dispels fear, alleviates misconceptions, and encourages people to fast in a sensible way. In this chapter we will answer five of the most common questions that we receive at our seminars:

1. I would like to fast, but I'm afraid I couldn't hold out. How do I overcome this fear?
2. What can I do to prepare for a fast?
3. How do I handle irresistible cravings to eat?
4. How should I break my fast?
5. What kind of diet should I pursue after a fast?

You may be asking yourself some of these same questions. Let's look at each one individually.

Conquer the Fear of Fasting

As earlier chapters explained, you must conquer the fear that fasting will harm your body. You won't starve to death while fasting. The information in this book should dispel any fears of fasting that you may have harbored.

The fear of fasting is one of the contraindications to fasting. Whether the fast is undertaken for spiritual or therapeutic reasons, fear can upset the emotional balance of the faster and can hinder the outcome. Having faith in fasting and maintaining emotional balance throughout the fast is so important that experienced natural hygiene practitioners never recommend fasting to those who are not willing. Why? Fear upsets the neurological, hormonal, physiological, and biochemical balance of the body and can—in extreme cases, whether fasting or not—result in death. Medical evidence shows that some people who have been cut off from food because of a natural disaster die prematurely—long before they reach starvation. They died, not from fasting, but from poisonous endogenous toxins that the body created out of an intense, chronic fear of being without food.

Because emotional balance contributes to the effectiveness of fasting, I advise people to prayerfully consider when they should fast. If your faith in fasting is strong, times of emotional turmoil may be the best time to rest in the Lord and fast. But if the emotional turmoil is too upsetting, you should probably continue eating regular meals until balance is restored. Generally speaking, I advise people not to fast when emotional turmoil burdens them. The following times bring additional stress:

1. The trauma of separation or divorce
2. The loss of a loved one
3. Pregnancy and nursing after giving birth
4. Stressful situations that cause anger, extreme anxiety, or any other intense emotional strain

Exceptions, of course, do occur. You need to be sensitive to the Holy Spirit to discern His will. Even though you may be suffering grief, stress, or intense emotional strain, God may still lead you to fast. How will you know? Ask yourself the following questions:

1. Have I received a special message from God to fast?
2. Have I reached a place of spiritual desperation and temporarily lost the desire for food?
3. Have I decided to fast for a specific health problem?

I hope this book has convinced you that you need not fear fasting. By now you should be gaining confidence in this neglected discipline. If you understand the following three points, you can conquer the fear of fasting:

1. Fasting does not harm our bodies. Moderate, sensibly conducted fasting actually benefits the body.
2. Most of us can fast many days, even several weeks, on the stored reserves in the body.
3. The body always signals when it's through fasting and requires food. Unless we go on the consecration or completed fast, we shouldn't be concerned about the transition from fasting to starvation.

With this knowledge, we can enter a fast free of fear so that we are psychologically ready for optimum results.

Preparing for Your Fast

How can you prepare spiritually for a fast? I think the best way is to fill your heart and mind with Scripture. Your body feeds on your reserves during a fast, but you must nourish your spirit. During a fast we understand that man doesn't *"live by bread alone"* (Matthew 4:4).

Fasting gives us an opportunity to deny the lusts of our flesh. During this time, we are no longer slaves of sin, in bondage to food. The old nature was crucified with Christ. We are "new creations" in Christ. (See 2 Corinthians 5:17.) Remind yourself of these spiritual truths during your fast.

Here are some of my favorite passages that I meditate on when fasting:

> *Walk in the Spirit, and you shall not fulfill the lust of the flesh. For the flesh lusts against the Spirit, and the Spirit against the flesh; and these are contrary to one another, so that you do not do the things that you wish.* (Galatians 5:16–17)

> *Be sober, be vigilant; because your adversary the devil walks about like a roaring lion, seeking whom he may devour.* (1 Peter 5:8)

> *Put on the whole armor of God, that you may be able to stand against the wiles of the devil.*
> (Ephesians 6:11)

> *Do not let sin reign in your mortal body, that you should obey it in its lusts. And do not present your members as instruments of unrighteousness to sin, but present yourselves to God as being alive from the dead, and your members as instruments of righteousness to God.*
> (Romans 6:12–13)

> *I will praise You, for I am fearfully and wonderfully made; marvelous are Your works, and that my soul knows very well.* (Psalm 139:14)

> *And whatever we ask we receive from Him, because we keep His commandments and do those things that are pleasing in His sight.*
> (1 John 3:22)

> *Therefore, whether you eat or drink, or whatever you do, do all to the glory of God.*
> (1 Corinthians 10:31)

> *My son, give attention to my words; incline your ear to my sayings. Do not let them depart from your eyes; keep them in the midst of your heart; for they are life to those who find them, and health to all their flesh.* (Proverbs 4:20–22)

How should you prepare physically for a fast? Because many people experience a great drop in their blood sugar when they forsake their usual high-fat, high-sugar diets, you may want to wean yourself from these foods a day or two before your fast. If you're a heavy coffee or tea drinker, gradually cut the caffeine from your diet. Fasters commonly experience headaches, a withdrawal symptom of forgoing their usual large amounts of caffeine and sugar. Eliminating these foods before the fast will decrease the likelihood of your suffering with headaches, dizziness, and cravings.

Overcoming Satan's Temptations

Just because you've decided to consecrate a fast unto the Lord, do not expect an easy task. Satan may attack you with great regularity and even greater force. Remember, you are being refined into spiritual gold through these attacks. Fear not! Use the Word of God as a powerful weapon against these attacks to stop the fast and raid the refrigerator.

If you've ever been tempted to eat during a fast, you're not the only one who has experienced the fiery darts of the Enemy. Let's look at a passage of Scripture on Jesus' temptation during His fast.

> *Then Jesus was led up by the Spirit into the wilderness to be tempted by the devil. And when He had fasted forty days and forty nights, afterward he was hungry. Now when the tempter came to Him, he said, "If You are the Son of God, command that these stones become bread." But He answered and said, "It is written, 'Man shall not live by bread alone, but by every word that proceeds from the mouth of God.'"...Then Jesus said to him, "Away with you, Satan! For it is written, 'You shall worship the* Lord *your God, and Him only shall you serve.'" Then the devil left Him, and behold, angels came and ministered to him.*
>
> (Matthew 4:1–4, 10–11)

Jesus underwent His consecration fast with the purpose of being tempted by the Devil and overpowering him! This is reason enough to fast unto the Lord—to claim victory over the Devil in your life so that you can better serve the Lord! Following His fast in the wilderness, Jesus entered into the most miraculous ministry the world has ever seen.

If the Devil had come to Jesus prior to His consecration fast and enticed Him with food, power, and self-glory, Jesus may have succumbed. But after consecrating His life to God through this extended fast, Jesus was not enticed by the earthly temptations that Satan dangled before Him. After all, it's never much of a battle when what the Tempter offers is not attractive! Although Jesus had not eaten for forty days and nights, His spiritual food sustained Him well—even through the onslaughts of Satan's temptations.

Jesus received rich rewards for overcoming temptation. Although He had performed no miracle before His fast, He immediately stepped into His new ministry. Jesus had God's greatest gifts at His disposal: the capacity to know what was in the hearts of men; the gift of teaching; the ability to heal, to cast out demons, and to perform miracles.

Since Jesus had not yet performed a single miracle, turning stones into bread could have been His first. He might have been anxious to use His new power. Knowing a lot about human nature, Satan wisely timed his appearance to Jesus because that could have been the most vulnerable moment in Jesus' life.

Satan cunningly challenged Jesus by using the word *if*. *"If You are the Son of God"* (Matthew 4:3). Jesus had just spent forty days fasting in intimate communion with God. During this time, Jesus realized His own divinity more than ever before. Jesus could have reacted with typical human pride by retorting, "What do you mean, *If* I am the Son of God? I'll prove it to you with My new miracle-working power!" Satan enticed Jesus to use His newly acquired power for a selfish reason and turn the stones into bread so that He could immediately break His fast.

Jesus could have turned the stones into bread. Furthermore, He could have succumbed to Satan's two other temptations. He could have cast Himself down from the pinnacle of the temple in Jerusalem, and the angels would have miraculously protected Him from harm. He could have accepted the offer of becoming the glorious ruler over earthly kingdoms if He would only fall down and worship Satan. Yes, Jesus could have succumbed to any one of these temptations. But He did not yield to His human nature. He had just consecrated Himself to God through fasting and prayer. He belonged only to God.

Satan hadn't anticipated that Jesus had completed this fast with indomitable, divine power on His side. In the face of Satan's cheap trickery, Jesus stood firm. He simply used the Word of God to vanquish the Devil: *"It is written, 'Man shall not live by bread alone, but by every word that proceeds from the mouth of God'"* (Matthew 4:4).

How do we meet with temptation while fasting? We must rely on the power of the Word during a fast to conquer the inevitable temptation by Satan. Our human willpower may work for the moment, but it is ultimately unreliable. Knowing this, Jesus quoted Scripture after the Devil attempted to lure Him away from God's plan.

The Word of God always defeats the Enemy in our own lives.

You can expect satanic attack during a fast. Satan tried to tempt Jesus during His fast, and he will try to tempt you. God's Word is our personal arsenal to stay on the fast. If we read God's Word, study it, memorize it; if we eat its spiritual food, if we drink it into our minds, emotions, and spirits, then we need not be tempted beyond our capacity to resist. Then we can say to Satan, "It is written...." We can meet with temptation, overpower Satan, and fast unto the Lord.

How to Break Your Fast

Let's suppose you've fasted unto the Lord. You met Satan head-on with the Word of God when he tempted you to raid the refrigerator. Now you are ready to break your fast—sensibly, moderately, and thankfully! How do you do it?

You can choose one of two ways. Either one is as good as the other. If you experience no digestive problems upon eating again, your decision is merely a matter of personal preference. Let's look at your choices.

1. *You may take juices.* On the first day, take four ounces of fresh juice every two hours, starting at 8:00 A.M. and ending at 6:00 P.M. On the next two or three days, take 8–10 ounces of freshly made juice for breakfast, lunch, and dinner.

Some people prefer juices because they are easy to digest and they don't present the temptation to overeat on solid foods. The juices may be freshly squeezed citrus juice or any kind of fresh fruit and/or vegetable juice made in a juicer. Usually, it is best not to mix the fruit with the vegetable juice, although carrot, apple, and celery juices are a very popular mix at hygienic retreats. Orange juice is undoubtedly the most popular. But fabulous juices made out of foods you would not normally think to juice—such as watermelon or tomato—are also wonderful choices.

2. *You may take fruit.* On the first day, take an eight-ounce serving of fresh fruit every two hours, starting at 8:00 A.M. and ending at 6:00 P.M. Eight ounces usually amounts to a single piece of fruit. With cantaloupe or apricots, you would have to actually weigh the fruit. On the next two to three days, take two to three pieces of fresh fruit (or the equivalent in larger pieces of fruit) for breakfast, lunch, and dinner. As with breaking a fast on juice, the orange seems to be the most popular food. Watermelon is also frequently chosen. Because all fruits are easy to digest, however, you may chose your favorite over the traditionally used foods for breaking your own fast. Be sure to eat slowly and chew your food well.

The Genesis 1:29 Diet

Let's assume that you've fasted successfully, you've broken your fast correctly, and you're now ready to resume a regular meal schedule. Instead of going back to the standard American diet, you may want to go on the partial fast of the Genesis 1:29 diet.

If we eat only natural, whole, unprocessed fruits, vegetables, nuts, and seeds served in their original, sun-cooked state, and if we abstain from all other foods, this is a partial fast. This is actually God's original diet handed down for the human race from the Garden of Eden!

> *And God said, "See, I have given you every herb that yields seed which is on the face of all the earth, and every tree whose fruit yields seed; to you it shall be for food."* (Genesis 1:29)

Other translations encourage us not only to undergo a partial fast from all animal products, but also to take our foods sun-cooked in their whole and natural state, just as nature serves them. God's original diet is identical to the diet originally proposed by the natural hygienist pioneers, nearly all of whom were Christians. The Genesis 1:29 diet and the natural hygiene diet are both identical to what God presented as our food plan in Genesis.

Scientific studies and statistical evidence now show that this totally vegetarian food plan of natural, whole, uncooked foods is also the ideal diet for superlative health, a feeling of well-being, and longevity. These studies should not surprise Christians. We know that God created man and woman. Is it any wonder that He left them with the perfect foods for perfect health?

These foods are nutrient-rich in all the necessary vitamins and minerals. They supply all the protein, carbohydrates, and fatty acids necessary for vibrant health. Because of the high water content of fruits and vegetables, they are 70 to 96 percent water. The foods are so water-sufficient that you probably won't require anything else to drink. If you do get thirsty, drink only freshly made juices or distilled water. Filtered or bottled water may be taken if you can't get distilled.

The Genesis 1:29 diet (God's ideal diet, also called the natural hygiene diet) is not only nutrient-rich and water-sufficient; it is also the ideal diet for disease-proofing your body. Here are some benefits of this diet:

1. Low in saturated fat
2. Virtually free of cholesterol
3. Does not overload the body with toxic protein
4. Free of toxic animal products
5. Rich in live enzymes
6. Calorie sufficient, but not too caloric for maintaining your healthiest weight
7. Fiber rich
8. Free of refined sugar and refined flour
9. Salt free
10. Caffeine free
11. Free of toxic chemical additives
12. Properly combined for easy digestion
13. Alkaline in metabolic reaction so that the calcium reserves are not depicted to neutralize acid wastes
14. Nontoxic, which means that it's easy to digest, it conserves nerve energy, and it doesn't drain the body of nerve energy like a toxic diet does

When the Genesis 1:29 ideal diet is part of a total health program that observes God's natural laws of health, including fasting, this is as close to "God's health insurance" as we can come!

We use this food plan in our Genesis 1:29 conferences where we serve groups of people over a period of one to two weeks. You'll see that a vast variety of foods is available on this wonderful health program. One need never be bored on this diet. God gave us a wealth of ideas for our menu planning.

Having had a difficult time of eating a nutritious diet on her own, one of our Born Again Body conference attendees was delighted to learn God's proper eating program. As she gazed over our bountiful dinner buffet, she turned to me and marveled, "Lee, I just couldn't imagine all this. I had a hard time thinking past a lettuce and tomato salad!" The following menus represent the diet promoted by our Born Again Body Spa program.

Born Again Body Typical Menus

On this program, you can enjoy three wholesome, satisfying meals each day. Allow several hours between meals. Nothing should be taken between meals except distilled water, and this only thirty minutes after fruit meals, two hours after starch meals, and four hours between protein meals, or at least fifteen minutes before eating.

We encourage the attendees at our Born Again Body conferences to eat fruit for breakfast. This helps to cleanse the body and start the digestive system functioning after breaking its fast from the previous night. A tropical delight breakfast welcomes our conferees each morning. The breakfast buffet has three sections:

1. Fresh fruit (a half dozen or more varieties)
2. Soaked, dried fruit (one or two varieties)
3. Dried fruit (two or three varieties)

Your breakfast can vary according to the availability of fruit in your area of the country. Fruit is best when eaten in its natural, raw, whole state. By cutting the fruit as it is eaten, you will preserve the nutrients until you consume them. Fruit should be stored in cool, dry place and served at room temperature for optimum flavor When fruit must be refrigerated, it should be brought to room temperature before serving.

We discourage people from using condiments on their foods and drinking liquids during meals. At our health conferences we keep a pot of hot distilled or filtered water available for those who feel they must drink something with their meals. You may want to flavor yours with a slice of lemon or lime. Cold distilled or filtered water is a good choice for a beverage. Tap water should not be taken—only filtered, distilled, spring, or well water.

Tropical Delight Breakfast

1. *Fresh fruit:* Our southern California climate affords us a variety of fresh fruit throughout the year. Here are some of the choices we enjoy at our tropical delight breakfast:

Large Mexican papaya: served whole on large platter with large kitchen knife for cutting.

Watermelon: served same as Mexican papaya.

Melons: a variety of cantaloupe, honeydew, and so on. Seeded, halved, or if very large, quartered.

Pineapple: peeled and sliced into circles about one-half inch thick. Served on platter with large fork.

Grapefruit: preferably the smaller variety. Served whole, piled high on large platter.

Oranges: served same a grapefruit, whole.

Apples: different varieties. Served same as citrus.

Small seasonal fruit: tangerines, plums, peaches, grapes, strawberries, and so on. Served whole. (Berries should not be stemmed.)

Limes and/or lemons: halved or quartered (a must for every buffet).

2. *Soaked, dried fruit:* prunes, apricots, and so on. Only one kind on each morning buffet. Soaked overnight in hot (not boiling) water. Served in a large bowl near a stack of individual sauce dishes.

3. *Dried fruit:* A variety of two or three, such as peaches, dates, and pineapples.

Lunch

Soup of the day (non-creamed): Chef's choice made with no animal products. Examples offered in Appendix 2.

Prepared salad: Chef's choice such as slaw, Waldorf, carrot, tossed, and so on. The prepared salad sometimes includes fruit, which is the only exception on the all-vegetable lunch buffet.

Salad bar: list follows.

Salad dressings: always the same for lunch and dinner. List follows.

Soft, hot corn tortillas served in covered baskets or a multi-grain bread.

Note: We encourage our conference attendees to refrain from using salt, pepper, sugar, or cream.

Salad Bar

Lettuce: a variety is preferable, served whole. Each kind served on separate platter with serving tongs. (No iceberg lettuce, please.)

Spinach and/or other salad greens: served same as lettuce.

Watercress: served same as lettuce.

Celery: large, individual stalks, served whole.

Carrots: preferably the small, tender variety: served washed but unpeeled. They can be cut crosswise into two- or three-inch pieces or grated and served on serving plates with serving fork or small tongs.

Jicama, zucchini, beets, or other appropriate raw vegetables: served cut in sticks, sliced, or grated as with carrots.

Cucumber: washed, unpeeled, cut crosswise into large (two- to three-inch) pieces.

Tomatoes: preferably the smaller variety. Served whole, piled high on platter.

Avocados: preferably the smaller, miniature variety. Served whole, but cut into four sections. Note: Keep together to prevent turning brown.

Sprouts: various kinds.

Green onion: served whole.

Cabbage, green and/or red: grated.

Radishes: served whole with stems, unless stems look old; then they should be trimmed.

Hot chilies

Salad Dressing Ingredients

We serve these at the end of our raw salad bar. Small sauce dishes or cups are usually available for those who want to mix the various ingredients for their own individual salad dressing. This section should always be the same for lunch and dinner.

Mexican salsas can be made in two ways. The first uses fresh tomatoes and onions, finely chopped. Add a touch of cilantro, garlic, and lime juice. The second salsa is made the same as above, but with enough hot chilies to make sauce mildly hot.

Guacamole is made with avocados, grated onion, diced tomatoes, diced hot chilies, and small amount of cilantro for very mild taste. Mash and mix with a few drops of lemon juice and garlic juice.

Lemons and/or limes: Served halved or quartered, depending on size.

Olive oil

Almond oil or safflower

Pumpkins seeds, unsalted

Sunflower seeds, raw

Raisins

Vege-Base

Dr. Jensen's Seasoning

Gourmet Delight, four flavors

Dinner

(Combination Fruit and Vegetable Buffet)

1. Adam and Eve buffet is a smaller version of the fruit served at breakfast and the vegetable bar served at lunch. Start your meal with the fruit.

2. One non-starch vegetable casserole.

3. One starch. Prepared potatoes, baked potatoes, and yams, or rice, wheat, wheat pasta, or other selection.

4. Corn tortillas; brown, black, or sprout bread.

5. On each table: bowls of unshelled nuts (no peanuts) with nutcracker and bowl for shells.

By fasting on a regular basis, you can regain your lost health; by eating a nutritious diet between fasts, you can maintain it. After your body accustoms itself to this new way of eating, your energy level will soar, you'll cultivate a taste for natural foods, and many of your eating-induced health problems will disappear. What more could you ask for?

Sixteen

Closing Encouragements

I encourage you to fast unto the Lord, but I want you to do much more than that. Fasting will enrich your Christian life like few disciplines can. As a result of fasting, be open to deepening your commitment to the Lord and to pouring yourself out in service more than you ever imagined you could. Feeling close to God while fasting is wonderful, but the deeper commitment and the outpouring of service at the end of your fast are your true rewards.

Jesus Christ showed us how to fast unto the Lord. God launched His powerful ministry only after a prolonged fast. After His consecration fast in the wilderness, Jesus traveled to Galilee. There He taught in the synagogues, preached the Gospel, and healed all kinds of diseases. Following His fast, Jesus' commitment to serve God flowed like a saving, healing river to all those who would listen. His powerful life fulfilled the words of the prophet Isaiah:

> *The Spirit of the Lord GOD is upon Me, because the LORD has anointed Me to preach good tidings to the poor; He has sent Me to heal the*

> *brokenhearted, to proclaim liberty to the captives, and the opening of the prison to those who are bound; to proclaim the acceptable year of the* Lord*, and the day of vengeance of our God; to comfort all who mourn.* (Isaiah 61:1–2)

In His forty-day consecration fast, Jesus received an anointing that launched Him into the greatest ministry this world has ever known. Pouring out His infinite love and using His spiritual gifts, Jesus served humanity with every breath He breathed. Jesus simply lived out the heart of the fasting instructions in Isaiah 58.

> *Is it a fast that I have chosen, a day for a man to afflict his soul? Is it to bow down his head like a bulrush, and to spread out sackcloth and ashes? Would you call this a fast, and an acceptable day to the* Lord*? Is this not the fast that I have chosen: to loose the bonds of wickedness, to undo the heavy burdens, to let the oppressed go free, and that you break every yoke? Is it not to share your bread with the hungry, and that you bring to your house the poor who are cast out; when you see the naked, that you cover him?...If you extend your soul to the hungry and satisfy the afflicted soul.* (Isaiah 58:6–7, 10)

God rewarded Jesus openly for fasting and praying in secret. His fast exemplifies the unconditional rewards that God has in store for those who fast unto Him. If you have ever longed to be free of petty selfishness, if you have ever yearned to overflow with love for a suffering humanity, if you have ever despaired for the needy but were unable to reach out from your complacency, if you have ever desired to eliminate your spiritual bankruptcy and truly become a fulfilled servant of God—then fasting in consecration and unconditional surrender is for you.

Separating Sheep from Goats

The true test of righteousness—separating the sheep from the goats—is our unconditional outpouring of love as we meet the desperate needs of others. Jesus' parable (see Matthew 25:31–46) suggests that we will be judged in the presence of all humanity. There will be those present to whom we have given what aid we can. But there will also be those whom we have neglected or held in contempt. Let's look at the entire passage.

> *When the Son of Man comes in His glory, and all the holy angels with Him, then He will sit on the throne of His glory. All the nations will be gathered before Him, and He will separate them one from another, as a shepherd divides his sheep from the goats. And He will set the sheep on His right hand, but the goats on the left. Then the King will say to those on His right hand, "Come, you blessed of My Father, inherit the kingdom prepared for you from the foundation of the world: for I was hungry and you gave Me food; I was thirsty and you gave Me drink; I was a stranger and you took Me in; I was naked and you clothed Me; I was sick and you visited Me; I was in prison and you came to Me." Then the righteous will answer Him, saying, "Lord, when did we see You hungry and feed You, or thirsty and give You drink? When did we see You a stranger and take You in, or naked and clothe You? Or when did we see You sick, or in prison,*

and come to You?" And the King will answer and say to them, "Assuredly, I say to you, inasmuch as you did it to one of the least of these My brethren, you did it to Me." Then He will also say to those on the left hand, "Depart from Me, you cursed, into the everlasting fire prepared for the devil and his angels: for I was hungry and you gave Me no food; I was thirsty and you gave Me no drink; I was a stranger and you did not take Me in, naked and you did not clothe Me, sick and in prison and you did not visit Me." Then they also will answer Him, saying, "Lord, when did we see You hungry or thirsty or a stranger or naked or sick or in prison, and did not minister to You?" Then He will answer them, saying, "Assuredly, I say to you, inasmuch as you did not do it to one of the least of these, you did not do it to Me." And these will go away into everlasting punishment, but the righteous into eternal life. (Matthew 25:31–46)

One day we will hear the truth that will separate obedient sheep from the renegade goats. What will make the difference? Not attending church, but feeding the hungry and giving drink to the thirsty. Not repeating creeds and doctrines, but sheltering the stranger and clothing the poor. Not speaking empty words of self-righteousness, but visiting the sick and imprisoned. As the parable reveals, only those who acted out of God's love for humanity will *"inherit the kingdom prepared for* [them] *from the foundation of the world"* (verse 34).

Who, then, was Christ Jesus? He was the simple, humble Son of God who spent His life in fasting and prayer; who taught the people and preached the Gospel of God; who fed the hungry and clothed the naked; who healed the sick and visited the imprisoned; who encouraged all whom He met to be strong in the Lord God Almighty.

And just where is Jesus Christ today? He is among us. He promised that whoever receives a little child in His name, receives Him. Whoever feeds the hungry or gives drink to the thirsty is with Him. Whoever takes in a stranger or gives clothing to the poor is with Him. Whoever visits the sick or those in prison is with Him. He is available to us whenever we reach out to others with the love of God.

Thy Will Be Done

Jesus Christ uses men and women to do the Father's will in this world. We can do nothing greater, therefore, than consecrate ourselves into the hands of God to recreate this world according to His plan.

In the Sermon on the Mount, Jesus Christ not only taught how best to give, pray, and fast. He also taught exactly what to pray:

> *Our Father in heaven, hallowed be Your name. Your kingdom come. Your will be done on earth as it is in heaven. Give us this day our daily bread. And forgive us our debts, as we forgive our debtors. And do not lead us into temptation, but deliver us from the evil one. For Yours is the kingdom and the power and the glory forever. Amen.* (Matthew 6:9–13)

In the Sermon on the Mount, Christ outlined the constitution and the bylaws for His kingdom. He described the blessings, responsibilities, requirements, and strategies. He gave specific instructions on giving, praying, and fasting. We must share this vision if His plan—to make the kingdom of God here on earth as it is in heaven—is to be fulfilled.

We must take our rightful places in God's kingdom to do our part to the best of our ability. God's kingdom is made up of people totally dependent on Him and completely interdependent on each other. There is no room for self-seeking, self-worshiping renegades and outlaws in God's kingdom.

We feel the reality of God's kingdom *"on earth as it is in heaven"* (Matthew 6:10) when we respond to crises in the lives of others. We hear of a flood in Missouri, starvation in Africa, an earthquake in El Salvador, and the fire-destroyed home of a mother and five children on welfare in our hometown. Our hearts may ache at these tragedies, but then we respond with contributions. And the world responds with relief money and relief crews. Something of the Spirit of God triggers this loving, life-saving response in us, among Christians and non-Christians alike. Heartfelt knowledge of human suffering has a way of breaking through the self-centered consciousness of cruel, cold, competitive life. God's Spirit expresses itself through those of us who reach out to the less fortunate, broken members of society.

Final Words

Fasting allows us to present our bodies *"a living sacrifice, holy, acceptable to God"* (Romans 12:1). We put to death our sinful desires so that we can more perfectly fulfill God's will in our lives. As we yield ourselves to God, He gives us a sense of belonging to His great kingdom. This belonging joins us to a mighty army.

We come out of our fast with the full knowledge that even our most humble works bear the stamp of God's love and approval. With that stamp comes a sense of universal fellowship. We have enlisted in God's holy army to serve in whatever capacity He presents. Whether God leads us to feed the hungry, clothe the needy, or bring the destitute into our homes, we do it for the least of His—and we will be well rewarded.

The final test of our faith is not found in the answer to "What have I achieved or what have I believed?" Instead, the answer to "How have I shown God's love to humanity through my everyday actions?" reveals our depth of commitment and outpouring of service.

If this desire is not the overpowering passion of your life, I encourage you to enter a time of serious fasting and prayer so that you might receive a clearer vision of how to serve humanity and minister to this desperate world.

> *It is God himself who has made us what we are and given us new lives from Christ Jesus; and long ages ago he planned that we should spend these lives in helping others.* (Ephesians 2:10 TLB)

God Himself will give you the grace to enter this time of prayer and fasting in such a way that you're *"not doing your own ways, nor finding your own pleasure, nor speaking your own words"* (Isaiah 58:13).

Appendix 1

Testimonies

After reading this book, you may agree that the healings I received during my fasts were nothing short of miraculous. But I'm not the only one who has experienced dramatic results through fasting. During my years of traveling and speaking on this topic, I've collected testimonies from people who have been healed as a result of fasting and maintaining a nutritious diet. Here are some examples.

Caffeine Deliverance

> The Lord has completely delivered me from caffeine! I had tried for twenty-five years on my own, but nothing worked. An aunt had started me on coffee when I was nine years old, but recently the excessive caffeine (over ten cups a day—not to mention tea, chocolate, and an occasional cola) had begun to cause stomach burning and irritability.
>
> I realized coffee was my idol. It was all I could think about. I even got out of bed during the night to make a pot just to satisfy my craving. But praise God! Through prayer and fasting, He's

healed and delivered me! I also used to have unbearable soreness, pain, and swelling in my breasts before my period. Since God delivered me from caffeine—no more problem.

—Nancy from Michigan

Kidneys Healed

Since I purchased your tapes on fasting and attended the breakfast when you spoke, I have been fasting—and God has been doing some mighty miracles. I have been healed of a kidney disease I have had since childhood. I can't begin to tell you all the Lord has done for me since you left.

—Debbie from Alaska

Multiple Healings

I was having almost constant headaches. I decided to quit taking Tylenol or aspirin every two hours. It wasn't that effective, and the Holy Spirit showed me that I was poisoning myself. I also started eating raw foods. There were some very rough days, but thanks to your tape series and the books I began to read, I stayed on the diet twelve days, then distilled water for two days. Here is a list of symptoms that are almost 100 percent gone: headaches, backache from neck to mid-back, constipation, constant urination, sinusitis, and hypoglycemia. Praise the Lord!

—Janet from Colorado

I have good things to report! My internist was amazed at the results of the fast. He said in all the years he's treated me, he's never seen me look so good. He was shocked to learn I had completely gone off the anti-depressant medication that he thought would be a lifetime treatment. He was pleased to see me fourteen pounds thinner than my last visit. At the time I was eating nothing (I was constantly starved) and gaining weight. I happily report I now eat what I desire (within reason), and my weight remains stable. Even I can't believe it.

—Name Withheld

I have been healed of a tumor in my breast because God gave me the knowledge of good nutrition and fasting. After seven months of carefully selecting my food without chemicals and keeping a proper diet, I am very healthy. Because of my testimony, many people are changing their bad eating habits.

—Joan Marie Pirone

Medically Supervised Fasts

Do these testimonies sound like mere subjective opinion? Dr. Alan Goldhamer sent me the following cases where fasting was used in conservative medical treatment. Examinations and tests confirmed the severity of the ailments that plagued these patients. Fasting and good nutrition helped these people to alleviate their symptoms and regain good health.

Case 1

Female, age thirty-seven. Diagnosed with myasthenia gravis of one year's duration. Treated medically with neostigmine for six months. The symptoms included extreme weakness and dysarthria (difficulty speaking). Thymus removal was scheduled. Fasted for sixteen days. By day four of the fast, symptoms began to resolve. After eleven days of feeding a fruit- and vegetable-based vegetarian diet, the patient was free of symptoms. Follow-ups at six weeks, three months, six months, and one year showed excellent compliance and a complete resolution of symptoms.

Case 2

Thirty-one-year-old male. Blood was found in routine urinalysis. Diagnosis with kidney biopsy and clinical laboratory of acute glomerular nephritis. Creatinine levels .18, urea 10.0, E.S.R. 52. Kidney function tests consistent with approximately 60 percent of normal function. Patient refused drug therapy and was fasted for fourteen days. Patient was placed on a vegetarian, fruit- and vegetable-based diet and given detailed lifestyle modification program. Reexamination at one month revealed no significant change in kidney function. By three months, all blood and urine tests were essentially normal and kidney function tests were within normal limits. Creatinine .12, E.S.R. 8, and so on.

Case 3

Thirty-one-year-old female. Medical history included chronic constipation. No unassisted bowel movements (without laxatives) for over twenty years. The patient also experienced abdominal pain and bloating for ten years. Sigmoidoscopy revealed a rectal ulcer. The ulcer forced patient to wear rectal napkin to keep blood from soiling clothes. Colostomy suggested. By the fourth day of her ten-day fast, the bleeding had stopped. By the fifth day of feeding, the bowels were moving spontaneously without blood. The patient was placed on a therapeutic diet and at three months was free of constipation, abdominal pain, and bleeding.

Case 4

Forty-year-old female. Complaints included midcycle spotting, dysmenorrhea, breast tenderness, premenstrual depression, low back and neck pain. Diagnosis included an easily palpated five-centimeter uterine fibroid tumor and PMS. Lumbar strain and cervical joint dysfunction. The patient was treated with chiropractic manipulation of the neck and placed on a twenty-nine day fast followed by fifteen days on a therapeutic diet. The tumor was completely resolved by the twenty-eighth day of the fast. A three month follow-up revealed no recurrence of the fibroid tumor. Menstrual cycles had reestablished without PMS symptoms. There had been no neck or back pain since the fast.

Case 5

Fifty-five-year-old male. Acute pain in both hips on walking. Could not walk more than one hundred feet without pain. Diagnosis via angiogram of intermittent claudication due to severe atherosclerosis. Angioplasty surgery was recommended. The patient was placed on a therapeutic diet for six weeks and then fasted for twelve days. After the fast a progressive exercise program was instituted. Within one week of the fast, the patient was able to walk over two miles, including hills, without pain. A three-month follow-up revealed an apparent resolution of all claudication symptoms.

If you experience some amazing results with fasting, I would love to hear from you. Please send your testimony to the address listed on the copyright page of this book.

Appendix 2

Recipes

Now that you've heard about the amazing benefits of fasting and eating a nutritious diet between your fasts, you may be interested in altering your own eating habits. How can you make your meals appealing, tasty, and nutritious? Here are some of the favorite recipes I've collected over the years.

Fresh from the Garden

Raw Vegetable Salad:

Arrange on a plate 1 small head Boston lettuce; 2 medium-sized tomatoes, quartered; 1/2 green pepper; one cucumber, cut into 4 sticks; and 1 celery stalk.

Spinach Salad

4 cups spinach leaves, washed and dried
1/2 cup alfalfa sprouts
1/2 cup raw grated carrot

Place spinach leaves in a large salad bowl and garnish with sprouts and carrots.

Apple Green Salad

1/4 cup cashew butter (substitute with peanut butter)
Juice from 2 large lemons or limes
4 tsp. soy sauce substitute
1/8 cup safflower oil
1/4 cup water (or enough for a thin sauce)

Mix; then toss with Romaine or leafy green lettuce, raisins, walnuts, and green apples (halved, cored, unpeeled, and sliced).

Carrot Salad

Grated carrots, diced fresh pineapple, nuts, raisins with lemon, brown sugar or honey, and peanut butter.

Shangri-La Kidney Bean Salad

(Serves 3)
1 1/2 cups cooked kidney beans
1/4 cup chopped celery
1/4 cup chopped onion
1/4 cup chopped green pepper
1 tbsp. Dr. Jensen's Seasoning, Vegit, or Spike
(found in health food stores)
2 tbsp. safflower oil

Stir well and serve on lettuce leaf.

Asparagus Salad

(Serves 2)
2 lbs. fresh asparagus (or substitute frozen)
4 oz. raw pumpkin seeds (or substitute chopped or slivered almonds)

4 leaves Romaine lettuce
2 lg. or 4 sm. tomatoes
1 lg. or 2 sm. stalks bok choy
1 grapefruit (optional if tomatoes aren't very tasty)

Asparagus may be used either raw or cooked (or a combination of the two). Use only the tasty tender tips of raw asparagus (or as much of the asparagus stalk as you like raw). Taste-test it. If you use the asparagus cooked, cut off the tough and discolored bottom ends of the stalks and steam the tender ends for 2–3 minutes, taking care not to overcook. You may use the tender tips raw and then steam the more fibrous (but not tough) portions and use both in your salad.

Cut up asparagus and place in a large mixing bowl with pumpkin seeds or almonds. Wash, dry, and cut or break up Romaine lettuce into large bowl; wash and cut up tomatoes into bowl. Wash celery and bok choy; dice coarsely, and add to bowl. If your tomatoes are not very tasty, you may halve and juice a grapefruit and add its juice to your salad. Mix well and then chop up a bit with a paring knife to further blend ingredients.

Vegetable Favorites

Shangri-La Cole Slaw

(Serves 3)
1/2 head of cabbage (small), shredded or chopped
1/4 cup chopped green pepper
1/4 cup chopped celery
1/4 cup chopped onion
1 tsp. Dr. Jensen's Seasoning

2 tbsp. safflower oil
Lemon

Toss all together.

Mixed Salad

1 medium head Romaine lettuce
1/2 head Boston lettuce
1 cup slivered raw broccoli
1/2 ripe red pepper, thinly sliced
1/2 cup raw cauliflower, thinly sliced

Toss ingredients together in a large wooden bowl. Dress with 3 or 4 tbsp. cold pressed oil and 1 or 2 tbsp. vege-base (optional).

Carrots & Celery Shangri-La

(Serves 3)
2 cups carrots, sliced 1/8 to 1/4 inch
2 cups celery, sliced diagonally, 1/8 to 1/4 inch
1 tbsp. Vogue Vege-Base, if desired
1/4 cup cold pressed safflower seed oil

Combine all ingredients, except oil, and place in large bowl. Place on Shangri-La steaming trivet in pan, which has a tight-fitting lid, with enough water so that the surface of the trivet is above water. Bring water to boil, then reduce heat to keep steaming until tender but not mushy—about one hour, depending upon your taste and preference. Add oil just before serving.

Serve after large finger salad with one of the starch casserole dishes, such as potato. If another vegetable is served, it should be one of the steamed greens, such as broccoli or turnip greens. This is a mildly starchy dish, so proteins or tomatoes should not be served at the same meal.

Shangri-La Okra Casserole

(Serves 3)
1 lb. okra, washed and cut crosswise in 1-inch slices
1/4 cup chopped onion
2 chopped tomatoes
2 tbsp. safflower oil
Dr. Jensen's Seasoning to taste—approx. 1 tsp.

Lightly sauté chopped onion in oil. Add the sliced okra pods; cook 5 minutes. Then add chopped tomatoes. Simmer 15 minutes or until okra is done. Season with Dr. Jensen's Seasoning.

Shangri-La Sautéed Vegetables

(Serves 3)
Your choice of thinly sliced carrots, zucchini, onions, green peppers, or celery. Any greens can be sautéed in their raw state. Potatoes, cauliflower, green leaves, and broccoli have to be blanched first for 10 minutes.

1 chopped onion
1 zucchini, sliced crosswise
1 green pepper, chopped
2 stalks celery, cut in 1/2-inch slices
2 tbsp. safflower oil

Lightly sauté one chopped onion in 2 tbsp. safflower oil. Add the zucchini, any vegetables, pepper, and celery. Stir frequently until fork-tender.

Vegetable Plates

Eggplant on Lettuce

(Serves 4 to 6)
1 medium eggplant
1 large ripe tomato, cored, peeled, and chopped
1/3 cup finely chopped onions
1/4 cup finely chopped parsley
4 tbsp. olive or safflower oil
Vegetable seasoning to taste (optional)
Juice of 1/2 lemon
1 tsp. honey
Several leaves of Bibb lettuce

In a preheated oven, bake the eggplant until soft at 350°. Peel eggplant, chop the flesh, then place it in a bowl. Drain excess juice from tomato and add to the eggplant. Add the remaining ingredients except the lettuce. Blend well and refrigerate for several hours. Arrange the lettuce leaves around the edge of a serving plate, and spoon the eggplant mixture evenly in the center of each leaf.

Red Cabbage with Nuts

4 cups shredded red cabbage
2 cups boiling water
1 lb. nuts, chopped
3 tbsp. margarine

Cook cabbage 3 minutes in boiling water and drain. Mix cabbage with nuts, water, margarine, Jensen's Seasoning, and vege-base. Arrange in oiled baking dish and bake in 375° oven for 30 minutes.

Vegetable Stew Shangri-La

(Serves 3)
3 cups tomatoes, skinned and chopped to 1/2- to 3/4-inch pieces
1/4 cup bell pepper, chopped fine, 1/4 inch
3 tbsp. Dr. Jensen's Seasoning, or similar
2 cups celery, leaves and all, sliced diagonally into 1/8- to 1/4-inch strips
1 cup string beans, sliced diagonally into 1-inch strips
1 cup okra, capped and cut into 1/2-inch pieces
2 cups eggplant, peeled and cubed into 1/2- to 3/4-inch pieces
1/4 cup cold pressed safflower seed oil
Note: If eggplant is not available, zucchini may be used.

Place tomatoes, bell peppers, and seasoning in stainless steel or similar pan. Bring to boil and simmer over low heat for 15 minutes to reduce water content. Add celery, string beans, and okra. Simmer for another 15 minutes or until tender but not mushy. Turn off heat, add the eggplant, and let stand for 15 minutes. Mixture should be of thick stew consistency, not soupy. Add oil and serve after a large salad with steamed, non-starchy green vegetables. Since this is not a starch dish, fresh tomatoes may be served with the salad if desired. Carrots or other starchy foods should not be served for correct combining.

Gazpacho

(Serves 2)
4–5 large tomatoes
1/2 cucumber

1/2 green pepper
1 slice onion
6 tbsp. olive oil
3 tbsp. vinegar
1/2 tsp. black pepper
1/8 tsp. cumin seeds

Using blender or food processor, blend tomatoes, cucumber, green pepper, onion, oil, vinegar, black pepper, and cumin seeds until mixture is the consistency of soup. Chill. Serve with diced tomatoes, cucumber, and green peppers as condiments.

Bean Soup

(Serves 6 to 8)
1 1/2 cups dried navy beans, soaked overnight in 8 cups water
3 tbsp. olive oil
2 medium-sized onions, chopped
3 cloves garlic, crushed
1/2 cup fresh coriander, finely chopped
1 medium-sized carrot, finely chopped
1 large potato, cut in 1/2-inch cubes
3 large tomatoes, chopped
2 1/2 tsp. salt
1/2 tsp. pepper
1/4 tsp. allspice

Place the beans and the water in which they have soaked in a pot and cover. Cook over medium heat for about an hour, or until the beans are cooked but still firm. Heat the oil in a frying pan. Then add the onion, garlic, and coriander; sauté, stirring continually until they begin to brown. Add the frying pan contents and the remaining ingredients to the beans, then simmer until all the vegetables are well cooked.

Split Pea Soup

(original recipe from "Pea Soup Andersen's" restaurant)
2 qts. soft water
2 cups Andersen's specially selected green split peas
1 stalk of celery, coarsely chopped
1 large carrot, chopped
1 small onion, chopped
1/4 tsp. ground thyme
1 pinch of cayenne
1 bay leaf, Vogue Vege-Base and/or Dr. Jensen's Seasoning

Mix all ingredients together. Boil hard to 20 minutes, then slowly until peas are tender. Strain through fine sieve and reheat to boiling point. You're in for a treat! This is the one that made Andersen's nationally famous.

Dress Up with Sauces

Honey Nut Dressing

1/2 cup cold pressed safflower or almond oil
1/4 cup raw, unsalted cashews
1/4 cup water
3 tbsp. honey
1 tbsp. fresh lemon or lime juice
2 tbsp. distilled white vinegar (or substitute for more lemon juice)
1 1/2 tsp. dried dill weed

3/4 tsp. light soy sauce (or salt-free soy sauce substitute)

Mix all ingredients in blender until very smooth. Store in jar in refrigerator. Toss with Romaine leaves, green leaves, leafy green lettuce, spinach, small orange pieces, and raisins. Yields 1 1/4 cups.

Mustard Dressing

1/2 cup water
1/4 cup unsweetened grapefruit juice concentrate
2 tbsp. mild Dijon-style mustard
1/2 tsp. curry powder

Thoroughly mix ingredients for dressing and toss with fruit and vegetables before serving.

Fresh Mexican Salsa

8 large tomatoes, coarsely diced
1 large onion, peeled and finely chopped
2 cloves garlic, peeled and minced
2 tbsp. chopped parsley
2 tbsp. chopped cilantro (optional)
1/4 to 2 tsp. chopped jalapeño chili, to taste

Combine all ingredients and toss gently. Yields 5 cups.

Marinara

4 tsp. olive oil
1 cup finely chopped onion
1/2 cup finely chopped carrot
2 tsp. fresh basil

4 tsp. finely chopped parsley
1/2 bay leaf
2 lbs. fresh tomatoes, coarsely chopped
1 tbsp. tomato paste (salt-free)
Freshly ground pepper
Hot red pepper flakes (optional)

Cook onions in oil until translucent. Add carrots and cook 4 minutes. Add basil, parsley, and bay leaf; simmer 2 minutes. Add tomatoes, pepper, and tomato paste, and simmer 30 minutes. Add red pepper flakes, if desired. Yields 3 cups. (You may want to peel tomatoes for some dishes, such as pizza, because the peels definitely change the texture of the finished dish.)

Lemon Dressing

2/3 cup oil (cold pressed)
1/3 cup lemon juice
1 clove garlic, minced
1/2 tsp. prepared mustard
1 1/2 tsp. salt
1/4 tsp. pepper

Combine all ingredients in blender; blend 5 minutes. Store in covered jar in refrigerator. Yields 1 cup.

Basic "Peaches" Vegetable Salad Dressing

Adjust portions to taste: lemon juice, cold-pressed oil, permissible seasonings, soy sauce substitute (optional).

Banana Sandwiches

Lettuce

Bananas
Raisins or dates

Wash and dry lettuce leaves; peel and halve bananas; and slice banana halves lengthwise. Place banana slices down the middle of lettuce leaves and top with soaked or dry raisins and/or pitted dates. Drizzle with honey nut dressing. Fold over each slice and eat like a sandwich. This requires manual dexterity, but the results are delicious!

Born Again Body Reducing Menus

Once you have broken a fast, you may want to avoid the standard American diet with its salt-filled, chemical-laden foods. You would benefit from going on a partial fast that permitted only the best raw fruits and vegetables. The following sample menu, which we recommend to post-fasters at our Born Again Body retreats and conferences, will also help you to pare down your weight.

Monday

Meal #1: One ripe banana, two red delicious apples.

Meal #2: Vegetable salad: four whole leaves of Romaine lettuce, four whole leaves of escarole, 1/2 cucumber, two stalks of celery, one small green pepper, two ounces of alfalfa sprouts, one medium-sized tomato, 1/4 avocado (three ounces).

Tuesday

Meal #1: Six ounces of concord grapes, two Bartlett pears.

Meal #2: Vegetable salad: four whole leaves of Romaine lettuce, four whole leaves of iceberg lettuce, two ounces of alfalfa sprouts, 1/2 cucumber, one small red bell pepper, three stalks pascal celery, one medium ripe tomato, and two ounces raw, unroasted nuts.

Wednesday

Meal #1: One medium slice of watermelon (three pounds).

Meal #2: Vegetable salad: four whole leaves of Romaine lettuce, and four leaves of Boston lettuce, 1/2 cucumber, two ounces mung bean sprouts, two stalks of celery, one medium ripe tomato, one small green pepper, 1/4 medium avocado (three ounces).

Thursday

Meal #1: Two oranges, one medium grapefruit.

Meal #2: Vegetable salad: four leaves of Romaine lettuce and four leaves of Bibb lettuce, one small green pepper, three stalks celery, 1/2 cucumber. Steamed: four ounces asparagus, one cup brown or wild rice (cooked).

Friday

Meal #1: One ripe banana, two golden delicious apples.

Meal #2: Vegetable salad: four whole leaves of Romaine and iceberg lettuce, one small green pepper, two stalks celery, one medium ripe tomato, 1/2 cucumber, four leaves of escarole, two ounces raw, unroasted unsalted nuts.

Saturday

Meal #1: Six ounces green seedless grapes, two mackintosh apples.

Meal #2: Vegetable salad: four whole leaves of Romaine and four whole leaves of Bibb lettuce, one small red bell pepper, three stalks celery, 1/2 cucumber, one medium ripe tomato, two ounces alfalfa sprouts, 1/4 medium avocado (three ounces).

Sunday

Meal #1: One cantaloupe (two pounds).

Meal #2: Vegetable salad: four whole leaves of Romaine lettuce, four whole leaves of Boston lettuce, 1/2 cucumber, one small green pepper, three stalks celery, four leaves escarole. Steamed: one four-ounce white potato steamed with skin on and then peeled before eating, four ounces turnip greens.

No condiments or seasoning of any kind are to be used on this program. This includes powders, cold pressed oils, lemon juice, vinegar, and so on. You may substitute similar fruit, depending on your preference and what is available in season in your area. Watch the pounds come off!

Appendix 3

Natural Hygiene

This appendix will give you more information on the physical benefits of fasting from a hygienic view. I want to thank Victoria Bidwell, whom I met at one of my Genesis 1:29 conferences, for compiling, organizing, and writing the following information. I also want to thank Vivian Vetrano, a medical doctor and one of the foremost natural hygienists of our time, for scrutinizing this material to make sure it is scientifically and hygienically correct.

The Basic Tenets of Natural Hygiene

1. Health, which is the normal state of all living organisms, is maintained through natural, self-initiating, self-healing processes.

2. The one cause of all disease is toxic saturation at the cellular level of the bodily tissues, bloodstream, and fluids brought on by the depletion of nerve energy reserves through wrong living habits. This state of self-poisoning is termed autointoxication, toxicosis, or toxemia.

3. Disease is retrograde change on the cellular level as a result of toxicosis. In order to prevent these changes and to forestall degeneration for as long as possible, the body attempts to isolate or eliminate abnormal accumulations of metabolic waste and ingested poisons. Such attempts at elimination may be called acute disease and serve to prevent these degenerative changes.

4. Because toxicosis is the one cause of all disease, natural hygiene refutes the concept that microorganisms, germs, or viruses are the sole cause of disease.

5. Because only the body is capable of instituting cleansing and healing processes, natural hygiene rejects the ingestion of substances that the body cannot metabolize and assimilate and that cannot be used in the normal, metabolic processes to be appropriated into bodily tissue. Such unnatural substances can only further enervate and poison the body and are not to be considered food or nutrition in any way. Both medication and "quasi-food" substances typical of the chemical-laden, processed food supply are included in this enervating, poisoning category and are, therefore, considered to be life threatening.

6. Natural hygiene recommends the following as the ideal diet and the only food fit for the highest level of human health and well-being: whole raw fruits, vegetables, nuts, and seeds prepared in proper combination and eaten in moderation when in a state of emotional balance.

7. Natural hygiene employs fasting, which provides deep physical, physiological, sensory, mental, and emotional rest. This deep and almost total rest provides the body with ideal conditions for the regeneration of nerve

energy needed for the repair of damages and for the elimination of toxins.

8. Health is the personal responsibility of each individual. Vibrant health is achieved only by conscientiously applying healthful living practices in all areas of one's life.

The One Cause of All Disease

According to natural hygienists, the one cause of all disease is toxemia, autointoxication, or toxicosis. These three words are almost synonymous for the one cause of all disease and low energy. As pointed out earlier, the dictionary definition of toxemia means poisons in the blood; it is sometimes used to mean a generalized state of autointoxication. But toxemia is a narrowly defined term in natural hygiene: toxemia refers specifically to the saturation of the bloodstream with toxic waste, caused by insufficient nerve energy to perform basic elimination tasks at the cellular level. By contrast, toxicosis refers specifically to the more advanced bodily condition of toxic poisoning, not only of the blood, but of the other bodily fluids and individual cells and the tissues themselves. Finally, autointoxication is a general term, simply meaning self-poisoning.

When nerve energy is low, elimination of toxic waste is impeded: the body must operate under a toxic handicap. Poisons saturate first the bloodstream and bodily fluids, and then the cells, tissues, organs, and system. The descent into disease begins.

Continued toxic overload results in a state of autointoxication throughout the blood, lymphatic fluids, and tissues of the body. Toxicosis affects the entire body.

The weaker organs feel the effects more strongly and break down first. A very vascular organ or an organ of elimination may take the brunt of many poisons that flow into the organ. In acute disease, the body may choose an avenue such as the lungs, nose, and sinuses to eliminate them. In degenerative disease, the overload may result in waste being stored in out of the way deposits: joints, arteries, fatty tissues, tumors, and cysts. In acute and chronic disease, the avenue of toxic elimination or the location of toxic deposits often determines the name of the disease given by the medical profession.

We auto-intoxicate ourselves in two ways: from within the body (endogenous toxemia) and from what we ingest from outside the body (exogenous toxemia). The true health seeker learns to minimize the former and almost totally eliminate the latter. We create endogenous toxins from:

1. Metabolic waste; ongoing, toxic by-products on the cellular level
2. Spent debris from cellular activity
3. Dead cells
4. Emotional and mental distress and excess
5. Physical fatigue, distress, and excess

We ingest exogenous toxins from:

1. Unnatural food and drink
2. Natural food deranged by cooking, refining, and preserving
3. Improper food combinations that result in endogenous toxins
4. Medical, pharmaceutical, herbal, and supplemental drugging

5. Tobacco, alcohol, and all forms of recreational drugging
6. Environmental, commercial, and industrial pollutants
7. Impure air and water

We can also enhance our energy reserves by living according to healthful practices. Here are lists of energy enhancers and energy robbers that we need to identify in our lives:

Energy Enhancers

1. Cleanliness—both external and on the level of the bodily tissues and fluids
2. Pure air
3. Pure water
4. Adequate rest and sleep
5. The ideal diet
6. Adequate sunshine and natural light
7. Right temperatures
8. Regular exercise
9. Emotional balance and freedom from addictions, with high self-esteem and a purposeful life
10. Nurturing relationships

Energy Robbers

1. Uncleanliness—both external and on the level of the bodily tissues and fluids..
2. Unclean air
3. Impure water
4. Inadequate rest and sleep

5. The standard American diet
6. Inadequate sunshine and natural light
7. Abnormal temperatures
8. Lack of regular exercise
9. Emotional imbalance and slavery to addictions, with low self-esteem and a purposeless life
10. Toxic relationships

To fully understand the importance of restoring high nerve energy in our lives, let's examine what happens when we drain—rather than restore—nerve energy. Dr. J. H. Tilden's revolutionary writing in the 1930s best explained what happens when "energy leaks" leave us enervated.

The Seven Stages of Disease

1. *Enervation:* Nerve energy is so reduced or exhausted that all normal bodily functions are greatly impaired, especially the elimination of endogenous and exogenous poisons. This begins the progressive and chronic process of toxemia toleration that continues through the following stages. The toxic sufferer does not feel his normal self. He feels either stimulated or depressed by the poisonous overload.

2. *Toxemia:* Nerve energy is too low to eliminate metabolic wastes and ingested poisons. These toxic substances begin to saturate first the bloodstream and lymphatic fluids and then the cells themselves. The toxic sufferer feels inordinately tired, run-down, and out of it.

3. *Irritation:* Toxic buildup within the blood and tissues and lymphatic fluids continues. The cells and tissues where buildup occurs are irritated by the toxic

nature of the waste, resulting in a low-grade inflammation. The toxic sufferer may feel exhausted, queasy, irritable, itchy—even irrational and hostile. During these first three stages, if the toxic sufferer consults a medical doctor for his low energy and irritability, the doctor tells him, "There's nothing wrong with you. These symptoms are 'all in your head.' You're perfectly healthy!"

4. *Inflammation:* The low-grade, chronic inflammation from stage three leads to the death of cells. An area or organ where toxins have amassed becomes fully inflamed. The toxic sufferer experiences actual pain, along with pathological symptoms at this point. With the appearance of these symptoms, the medical doctor finally gives the sufferer's complaint a name. Traditionally, medical scientists have named many of the 20,000 distinctly different diseases after the site where the toxins have accumulated and precipitated their symptoms. Once the symptoms are named, the doctor usually prescribes the antidote from his *Physician's Desk Reference* or from his memorized medical/pharmaceutical repertoire. Standard medical doctors begin drugging and treating at this stage.

5. *Ulceration:* Tissues are destroyed. The body ulcerates, forming an outlet for the poisonous buildup. The toxic sufferer experiences a multiplication and worsening of symptoms while the pain intensifies. Standard medical doctors typically continue drugging and often commence with surgery and other forms of more radical and questionable treatment at this stage.

6. *Induration (hardening or scarring of tissue):* Induration is the result of long-standing, chronic

inflammation with bouts of acute inflammation interspersed. The chronic inflammation impairs or slows down circulation. Because some cells succumb, they are replaced with scar tissue. This is the way we lose good, normal-functioning cells—by chronic inflammation and death of cells. Toxins may or may not be encapsulated in a tumor, sac, or polyp. The toxic sufferer endures even more physical pain, which is intensified by the emotional distress of realizing that he is only getting worse, regardless of his earnest, obedient, even heroic attempts to get well. Standard medical doctors continue with both drugging and surgery and all other kinds of procedures deemed appropriate, both conventional and experimental.

7. *Irreversible degeneration and/or cancer:* Cellular integrity is destroyed through their disorganization and/or cancerous proliferation. Tissues, organs, and whole systems lose their ability to function normally. Biochemical and morphological changes from the depositing of endogenous and exogenous toxins bring about degenerations and death at the cellular level. The toxic sufferer is a pathological mess: he is on his deathbed. Standard medical doctors declare at this stage, "There's no hope left. You don't have much longer to live. You need to set your affairs in order." Failure of vital organs eventually results in death.

Types of Disease

The terms *acute disease* and *chronic disease* are used throughout this appendix. These are very specific terms in the literature of natural hygiene. Their mutual exclusivity is best appreciated in the following:

Acute Disease

1. Has a short, sharp course of only a few hours, days, or weeks.

2. Has a relatively shorter period of development because of the body's lowered ability to tolerate toxic saturation. The acute sufferer may seem to flare up into the acute stage suddenly and with a great show of vitality.

3. May last only a few hours, days, or weeks after strict adoption of the energy enhancers and immediate abandonment of the energy robbers.

4. Reflects a strong enough supply of nerve energy and residual vitality that eliminating toxins and repairing tissues are still possible. (The body has sufficient vitality to conduct a healing crisis.)

5. Results in, at best, complete reversal of the disease process—if the energy enhancers are fully adopted and if the causes of autointoxication are removed.

6. Is designated remedial in nature, as acute disease is an orderly process by which the body attempts to detoxify and repair itself.

7. Uses nerve energy in the elimination of toxic waste and in cellular repair, such that tissue integrity and normal organ and systemic functioning are improved. The health seeker may feel enervated or exhilarated when the acute crisis is passed, depending on the amount of nerve energy expended and on the kind and amount of toxic overload expelled.

Chronic Disease

1. Persists for a long time—many months or years.

2. Has a relatively prolonged period of development because of the body's increased ability to tolerate toxic saturation. The chronic sufferer exhibits lowered vitality and experiences progressively worsening symptoms.

3. Will last the rest of the chronic sufferer's life if strict adoption of the energy enhancers and immediate abandonment of the energy robbers is not instituted.

4. Reflects a state of toleration of toxins: the body continues to eliminate toxins on a lower level than in acute disease. (In the latter stages of pathological conditions, especially after the use of medications for years, the chronic sufferer has a weak supply of nerve energy. Even in such a case, conducting the repair process is still possible—if the energy enhancers are strictly observed.)

5. Results in the complete arrest of the disease process and possibly in the reversal of much of the abnormal tissue changes and degenerations that have already taken place—if the energy enhancers are adopted soon enough and if the causes of autointoxication are removed.

6. Is remedial in nature if the energy enhancers are strictly followed. Some detrimental tissue changes, however, have taken place in chronic disease. The tissue degenerations are sometimes reversible, sometimes not—depending on the severity and the type of tissue damage.

7. Ends with cellular poisoning such that tissues, organs, and whole systems lose their functional integrity, ending in long-term misery and/or death of the chronic sufferer.

Fasting versus Starvation

Fasting in common usage is invariably confused with starvation. This inaccurate understanding of fasting is, therefore, the first misconception to clear up. Etymology, the study of word origins, sheds some light on these two terms.

Fasting is derived from the Anglo Saxon language, coming from the word *faest,* which means "firm" or "fixed." During these early periods of fasting, a person firmly withheld food from himself, fixed in his resolve not to eat. The word *starvation,* on the other hand, is derived from the Old English word *steorfan,* which means "pestilence" or "mortality." To starve meant to die, and that's what will happen if nutritional reserves are exhausted.

But as language evolved with all its local color, no doubt people who were famished from a day's work came to say, "I'm starving!" when they had gone only several hours without food. Please understand that fasting is not starvation! The following distinctions will clarify the proper usage of these words:

The Hygienic Fast

1. Occurs with complete abstinence from all food and nutrients while taking distilled water according to thirst.

2. Usually accompanied by a distinct lack of hunger.

3. Represents a peaceful period of rest willingly entered into and usually marked by a genuine calm.

4. Always undertaken for beneficial emotional, spiritual, or health reasons.

5. Properly supervised by a trained practitioner who daily monitors the faster's vital signs and subjective experiences.

6. Represents a process of the body utilizing its nutritional reserves and autolyzing morbid tissue while forgoing food.

7. Always followed by a time of supervised refeeding and feeling of increased well-being and improved health.

Starvation

1. May occur even while ingesting insufficient and nutrient-deficient amounts of food or may occur in the complete absence of food over any extended period of time.

2. Ordinarily accompanied by a strong sense of hunger.

3. Represents a torturous period of turmoil that is forced on the body by oneself (or by someone else) and marked by extreme distress.

4. Often undertaken for social, spiritual, or political coercion.

5. Never properly supervised.

6. Represents a process of the body—exhausted of its nutritional reserves—slowly breaking down its vital tissues.

7. Usually followed by learning to live with irreversible tissue damage; it is often followed by death.

Hygienic Fasting versus Just Not Eating

Now that the health seeker can no longer confuse fasting with starvation, let us make one more subtle distinction. Some people arrive at a hygienic school to undertake a so-called "fast" with bundles of work and reading material in which to absorb themselves during the long fasting days. They may spend full eight-hour workdays involved in these distractions. Such a fast does rest the digestive system and provide some benefits. But this is not a hygienic fast; it is just not eating. Remember: *rest is essential to fasting.*

Rest is defined as a period of inactivity during which the faculties can restore expended nerve energy. When we create wastes faster than the body can eliminate them and deplete our energies faster than the faculties can restore them, a period of rest and fasting enables the body to catch up, to houseclean, and to recharge its batteries. Dr. Shelton underscored this point in his delineation of the four kinds of rest secured during a fast. (The following list names five kinds of rest, separating emotional and mental rest.)

Five Kinds of Rest Needed while Fasting

1. *Physical rest:* The faster makes as few demands on his musculoskeletal system as possible and takes as much bed rest as possible He goes to bed to rest, relax, and sleep. Or he lounges around during his waking hours, securing as much physical rest as possible, interspersing his day with naps and then retiring early.

2. *Physiological rest:* During a fast, the tremendously energy-expensive process of digestion, assimilation, and elimination of food is halted. Physiologists

speculate that 70 to 75 percent of our nerve energy is spent on the daily processing of food. With fasting, however, the entire gastrointestinal tract—nearly the entire body—rests! The energy normally used to process food while eating is freed up to repair, restore, and renew the body, mind, and spirit. Although deep physiological rest is secured during fasting for most of the body, some organs and systems work overtime to carry out the many bodily activities listed below. The more toxic the individual, the more energy is needed to carry out these activities. That's why the faster must secure as much rest as possible on all levels.

3. *Sensory rest:* During a fast, the individual retreats from the sensory onslaught of day-to-day living. The faster should use his eyes, ears, and other sensory organs as little as possible and stay in a quiet place to secure a rest and respite for all the sensory organs.

4. *Emotional rest:* Ideally, the faster retreats to a hygienic school or retreat setting, away from all the emotional excitement of daily life. Since experts estimate that 90 percent of all illness is stress induced—although diet and lifestyle also play a role—this emotional rest is truly beneficial.

5. *Mental rest:* The faster puts away concerns and projects that demand mental effort and concentration. The brain is the housing for nerve energy. In order for the recharging that brings high health and energy to take place, the brain needs rest!

Four Bodily Activities during a Fast

Under these ideal conditions of proper rest, the body engages in healing processes that are, in fact, the reversal of the disease process detailed earlier under the seven stages of disease. Dr Shelton simplifies our grasp of fasting by recognizing four main bodily activities during fasting that contribute to the reversal of disease and the wondrous restoration of nerve energy.

1. Excess body fat is consumed; weight loss results.
2. Energy is diverted from digestive processes to other tissues where it is needed for repair and rejuvenation.
3. Deep physiological rest is secured for every organ and system of the body; nerve energy is restored, and the normal bodily functioning is resumed.
4. Breakdown of morbid tissue and elimination of waste occur. Deposits are broken down, and tumors are absorbed.

Other rejuvenating effects may and usually do occur during fasting. The skin color often becomes more youthful and acquires a better color and texture. The eyes clear up and become brighter. Normal physiological chemistry and normal secretions are reestablished. The mind is cleared and strengthened. The digestive tract empties itself of putrefied bacteria and decomposing food. Finally, the faster experiences surges of newfound, restored nerve energy!

Fasting Is Not a Cure

All of this sounds pretty marvelous—downright magical, in fact. At first the health seeker may have been skeptical after reading about fasting for health; now he may suddenly think he has discovered the panacea for everyone's ills flowing out of a veritable fountain of youth!

Please understand that the fast is neither magic nor a cure. The fast, in and of itself, does nothing! But the fast does provide all the ideal conditions under which the body best operates to heal itself. Remember the fifth basic tenet of natural hygiene: "Natural hygiene holds that only the body is capable of instituting cleansing and healing processes." The properly conducted fast, therefore, sets the stage and provides the props for healing. Then physical, physiological, sensory, emotional, and mental rest allow the body's innate healing powers to work expeditiously and within the limits of its vitality at the time of the fast.

To quote Dr. Shelton: "A properly conducted fast will enable the chronically ill body to excrete the toxic load that is responsible for the trouble, after which a corrected mode of living enables the individual to evolve into a more vigorous state of health."

The Healing Crisis

Whether fasting in cases of acute or chronic disease, the faster should be forewarned that if the elimination becomes profound, he may experience a healing crisis. It is not advisable—although it is sometimes necessary—to break the fast during a crisis. If it is not too expensive in nerve energy for the faster and if it does not endanger his life, it is advisable to fast until the period of acute discomfort is past and until the present elimination-and-healing process has run its natural course.

Most fasters experience no dramatic crises during their fasts. Some may experience one or two mild, fleeting incidents, which may run their course in an hour or two. The cleansing processes initiated by the fast are not usually of a violent or disagreeable nature. Most of the excretion of toxic materials is carried on without discomfort or inconvenience. Extremely toxic individuals, however, may expect to experience some discomfort, which is an indication that they were greatly in need of the fast.

Fasting in Chronic Disease

The time to fast is before a disease becomes chronic. Degeneration resulting from chronic toxemia takes places slowly, but it can progress to the seventh stage of chronic irreversible disease in any one of its many forms, including cancer. If a person fasts when his symptoms are in one of the first six stages of disease and he adheres to a healthier lifestyle, some pathological degeneration can be reversed. Much irreparable damage—even cancer—can be avoided.

All too often, however, the symptoms of acute illness are suppressed by overfeeding and drugging. The body is never allowed to eliminate its toxic overloads that have accumulated during years of wrong living practices. Because of this constant suppression and continuation of a toxic lifestyle, the person enters the seventh and final stage of disease. At this point, many people turn to fasting as a last resort. Because so much tissue damage may have already been done, patients may not be able to get well, let alone stay well.

In spite of all the abuses to which such a body has been subjected, beneficial results do occur through a fast. One important feature about fasting in chronic disease is the marked acceleration of detoxification that occurs. The body speedily frees itself of toxic overload. It is not uncommon for the long-standing symptoms to disappear or greatly subside. This often happens shortly after a healing crisis.

The Complete Fast

Hygienists often refer to the complete fast, in which the faster goes through various detoxification symptoms and perhaps a series of healing crises until the body has reached its highest possible state of purification at the cellular level. Typically, this takes four to five weeks. In some cases, however, the individual may not have enough reserves to fast this long and may have to undertake a series of fasts over a period of time to reach completion. To many health seekers, the complete fast is a dream to be fulfilled. The highest state of health, well-being, high energy, and mental clarity possible accompanies this purified state of the body.

What, then, are the signs of a completed fast? The primary signal given by the body that it's time to terminate a complete fast is the unmistakable return of natural hunger. The fast must never be prolonged after the body lets one know when its reserves are depleted. Eating must be resumed immediately! The following signs also accompany a completed fast:

- A bright, clear tongue (the once heavily coated tongue becomes clean and pink)
- Sweet breath, a fresh and clean-tasting tongue
- Normalized temperature

- Normalized pulse rate
- Normalized skin reactions
- Return to normal saliva flow
- A clear, light, odorless urine flow
- Odorless excreta
- Disappearance of acute symptoms of detoxification
- Resumption of normal pink color under the fingernails
- Increased rapidity with which blood flows back into the skin when forced out by pressure
- Disappearance of unpleasant body odor
- Bright, clear eyes that sparkle
- Renewed strength and vigor
- A feeling of joy and well-being

Not all these signs appear in every fasting case. Sometimes the tongue does not clear completely. But the return of natural hunger is the most obvious indication to the fasting supervisor that the faster's reserves are depleted and that the starvation period is beginning. At this point, the fast must be broken!

Repeated mention has been made of undertaking only a properly supervised fast. For the fullest rest and greatest healing to take place, the faster should go to a fasting retreat. For any health seeker deciding to take a fast of significant length, therefore, proper supervision by a trained specialist is necessary.

Fasting is sometimes difficult, but it is always enriching and rewarding. The names of a number of institutions that teach the principles of natural hygiene and offer supervised fasting as part of their educational program can be obtained through Lee Bueno's ministry. You should write for brochures ahead of time so that you may compare the types of facilities and programs offered.

Who Should Fast?

Now that we've defined fasting, how does the health seeker determine if he should fast, provided that time and money are available? We must keep in mind that Americans eat far more of the wrong foods than they should, exercise far less than needed, and rest far too little. These wrong living practices result in a buildup of unwanted waste material in the body and squander the supply of nerve energy. The script is set for the progressive tragedy of chronic, degenerative disease. According to this standard, therefore, virtually everyone could profit from undertaking a fast.

Dr. Shelton puts it even more directly:

> The time to fast is when it is needed. I am of the decided opinion that delays pay no dividends; that, due to the fact that the progressive development of pathological changes in the structures of the body with the consequent impairment of its functions does not cease until its cause has been completely and thoroughly removed. Putting off the time for a fast only invites added troubles and makes a longer fast necessary, if indeed it does not make the fast futile. I do not believe that any condition of impaired health should be tolerated and permitted to become greater. Now is the time to begin the work of restoring good health; not next week, next summer, or next year.

Who Should Not Fast?

While many people will benefit from a fast, some people should refrain from fasting. How do you know if you're in this category? Here are seven contraindications to fasting:

1. *Clients who are fearful of fasting.* Carefully planned, comprehensive education as to the purpose of the fast and what to expect can usually fully alleviate such fears that are, in reality, a holdover from the medical mentality and/or false interpretation of fasting as meaning starving.

2. *Clients who are extremely emaciated.* These persons may go on short fasts with definite benefit. With proper living between fasts, these people may be restored to health.

3. *Clients who are in extreme weakness or of extreme degeneration.*

4. *Clients who have inactive kidneys accompanied by obesity.* In such cases, the excess tissues loaded with toxic waste may be broken down faster than impaired kidneys are able to eliminate. The same may be said for a badly damaged liver—too many toxins can enter the bloodstream at once. Fasting in cancer of the liver and in cancer of the pancreas is especially to be avoided.

5. *Clients who have difficulty breathing because of heart disease, and clients with advanced stages of heart disease.* Caution must be taken with any abnormal rhythms of the heart.

6. *Pregnant women.*

7. *Clients taking insulin.*

For more information
on natural hygiene, write or call:

Victoria Bidwell
The HighJoy Homestead
c/o GetWell ★ StayWell, America
Box 558
Concrete, Washington 98237
(360) 853-7048
E-mail: victoriabidwell@aol.com
www.getwellstaywellamerica.com

Notes

Chapter 1

1. Simon, Gilbert I., and Harold M. Silverman, *The Pill Book* (New York: Bantam Books, 1979), pp. 545–547.

Chapter 4

1. Greenstone, Julius H., "Fasting and Fast Day," *The Jewish Encyclopedia,* ed. Isidore Singer, vol. 5 (1903), p. 347.
2. Ibid.
3. As cited by Joseph F. Wimmer, *Fasting in the New Testament* (New York: Paulist Press, 1982), p. 13.
4. Condensed from Oscar Hardman, "Fasting," *Encyclopedia Britannica,* ed. Walter Yust, vol. 10 (1952), p. 108.
5. Wimmer, pp. 13–22.

Chapter 5

1. Greenstone, p. 348.
2. Kell, C. F., and F. Delitzsch, *The Pentateuch,* from "Biblical Commentary on the Old Testament" (Michigan: William B. Eerdmans Publishing Company, 1956), p. 406.

Chapter 6

1. Carrington, Hereward, Ph.D., in *Fasting and Nutrition,* p. 490, as cited in *The Fasting Story II,* by Henry S. Tanner, M.D., et al. (Mokelumne Hill, CA: Health Research), p. 48.
2. Ibid.

Chapter 7

1. Kellog, J. H., "The Fasting Cure" in *Good Health,* January 1905, pp. 1–5, as cited in "Vitality, Fasting and Nutrition."
2. Tilden, John M., M.D., *Tumors* (1921), reprinted from Dr. Tilden's *Health Review & Critique* (Mokelumne, CA: Health Research).
3. "The Mazdazman," February 1906, p. 27.
4. Bragg, Paul, M.D., *The Miracle of Fasting* (Santa Barbara, CA: Health Science), p. 10.
5. Bragg, p. 64.
6. These experiments were reported in *The Fasting Story II* by Professor C. M. Child, Chicago University, from the experimental investigations in the Department of Zoology of the University of Chicago. Professor Julian Huxley began these experiments, and his son continued.
7. Bricklin, Mark, *The Practical Encyclopedia of Natural Healing* (Emmaus, PA: Rodale Press, 1976), pp. 174–175.
8. Ibid.
9. DeVries, Arnold, *The Therapeutic Fast* (Los Angeles: Chandler Book Company, 1963).

Chapter 8

1. Friedenburg, Dr. (noted physician from New York), as cited in *The Fasting Story II,* by Henry S. Tanner, M.D., et al. (Mokelumne Hill, CA: Health Research), p. 50.
2. Ibid.
3. Hume, Wilder, *History of Medicine,* as cited in *The Fasting Story II,* by Henry S. Tanner, M.D., et al. (Mokelumne Hill, CA: Health Research), p. 204.
4. Hotema, Hilton, *Fountain of Youth,* p. 45, as cited in *The Fasting Story II,* compiled in 1956 from the writings of Hilton Hotema by Health Research, Mokelumne Hill, CA, which was taken from "How to Fast Scientifically" by Otoman Zar-Adusht Hanish (Chicago: Mazdazman Press, 1912).
5. *The Fasting Story II* cites Professor Hilton Hotema's chapter on the "Law of Disease and Cure" in *Ancient Secret of Longevity,* in which he says that Mitchnikoff's research provided the first logical explanation in modern times of the degenerative changes that occur in the body—and why. Dr.

George W. Crile, Dr. James Empringham, and Dr. Alexis Cartel have confirmed his research.

6. Carrel, Dr. Alexis (famous biologist of the Rockefeller Institute), as cited in *The Fasting Story II* by Henry S. Tanner, M.D., et al. (Mokelumne Hill, CA: Health Research), p. 47.
7. Tanner, p. 43.
8. Tanner, p. 54.
9. Shelton, Herbert M., *Fasting Can Save Your Life* (Chicago, IL: Natural Hygiene Press).

Chapter 9

1. Most experts consider anyone who weighs 20 percent above the normal or desirable weight for his size as "clinically obese."
2. Bricklin.
3. Tarshis, Barry, *The Average American* (New York: Antheneum, 1979), p. 50.
4. Hyder, Dr. Quein Q., *Shape Up* (New Jersey: Fleming H. Revell, 1979), pp. 96, 98.

Chapter 11

1. Dake, Finis Jennings, *Dake's Annotated Reference Bible* (Lawrenceville, GA: Dake's Bible Sales), New Testament, p. 112, column 1; marginal reference letter *s.* "These Greater Works."

Chapter 14

1. Murphy, Cecil B., *Put on a Happy Faith* (Chappaqua, NY: Christian Herald Books, 1976), p. 10.
2. Some churches retain the symbolism of this by their Ash Wednesday services in which the priest marks their forehead. This begins a six-week period that, when understood in its highest sense, is one of contrition for sins.

Suggested Reading

Arndt, Rev. Herman, *Why Did Jesus Fast?* (Mokelumne Hill, CA: Health Research).

Bidwell, Victoria, *The Health Seekers Yearbook* (Fremont, CA: GetWell StayWell, America).

Bidwell, Victoria, *The Salt Conspiracy* (Fremont, CA: GetWell StayWell, America).

Bragg, Paul C., M.D. Ph.D., *The Miracle of Fasting* (Santa Barbara, CA: Health Science).

Cott, Allan, M.D., *Fasting: The Ultimate Diet* (New York, NY: Bantam Books).

DeVries, Arnold, *Therapeutic Fasting* (Los Angeles: Chandler Book Co., 1963).

Drummond, Henry, *The Greatest Thing in the World* (New Kensington, PA: Whitaker House, 1981).

Ehret, Professor Arnold, *Mucusless-Diet* (Beaumont, CA: Ehret Literature Publishing Co.).

Ehret, Professor Arnold, *Rational Fasting* (Beaumont, CA: Ehret Literature Publishing Co.).

Gross, Joy, *30 Days to a Born Again Body* (Secaucus, NJ: Lyle Stuart, Inc.).

Gross, Joy, *The Vegetarian Child* (Secaucus, NJ: Lyle Stuart, Inc.).

Josephson, Elmer A., *God's Key to Health and Happiness* (Old Tappan, NJ: Fleming Revell Co.).

Lovett, C. S., *Jesus Wants You Well* (Baldwin Park, CA: Personal Christianity).

McMillen, S. I., M.D., *None of These Diseases* (Old Tappan, NJ: Fleming Revell Co.).

Mendelsohn, Robert S., M.D., *Confessions of a Medical Heretic* (Chicago: Contemporary Books).

Oswald, Jean A., and Herbert M. Shelton, *Fasting for the Health of It* (Pueblo, CO: Nationwide Press, Ltd.).

Prince, Derek, *How to Fast Successfully* (New Kensington, PA: Whitaker House, 1995).

Prince, Derek, *Shaping History through Prayer and Fasting* (New Kensington, PA: Whitaker House, 1994).

Shelton, Herbert M., *Fasting Can Save Your Life* (Chicago: Natural Hygiene Press).

Smith, David R., *Fasting* (Ft. Washington, PA: Christian Literature Crusade).

Tilden, John H., M.D., *Toxemia* (Chicago: Natural Hygiene Press).

Wallis, Arthur, *God's Chosen Fast* (Ft. Washington, PA: Christian Literature Crusade).

Wimmer, Joseph F., *Fasting in the New Testament* (New York: Paulist Press).

About the Author

Lee Bueno is a conference speaker, author, composer, soloist, and evangelist, both overseas and in the United States. For close to thirty years, she and her late husband, Elmer, conducted major evangelistic crusades in Latin America, establishing churches using their own portable, inflatable building. The building was two-thirds the size of a football field and seated 3,000 people. They called it "La Catedral de Air," or "The Air Cathedral."

Lee has recorded nine albums both in English and Spanish. For three years, she was a regular soloist on the PTL Club in Charlotte, North Carolina, and more recently she traveled as a soloist for the Benny Hinn Crusades. She was a featured soloist on over 400 "Buenos Amigos" ("Good Friends") Spanish programs, hosted by her husband and produced by her son, Chris. These programs helped them to pioneer Christian television in more than sixteen Latin American countries on 200 stations, drawing an audience of 25 million viewers every week and bringing the Gospel into the privacy of the Latin home.

More recently, Lee's focus is on public school teachers both in Latin America and the U.S. Using a Teacher of the Year award event called "Celebracion Buenos Amigos," or "Good Friend Celebration," the educators are invited to join Lee as honored guests where gifts and awards are given as part of an evangelistic outreach to the teachers. The program includes the distribution of *El libro de Vida,* or *The Book of Hope,* containing the stories of Jesus and 100 questions for an open-book quiz.

Lee continues to travel in full-time ministry using her vocal talents and inspirational speaking to challenge Christians in their walk with God.

Product Information

For information on suggested books, teaching cassettes, and other materials, please ask for our Born Again Body catalog. We also have a listing of natural hygienists and natural hygiene retreats.

Information on our very own Born Again Body Hideaway in California is also available. For those unable to attend, we offer Genesis 1:29 home training, a great program that teaches you how to shop, cook, and eat a nutritious diet for the best health results. To receive information on any of these items, write or call:

Born Again Body, Inc.

P.O. Box 1675

Temecula, CA 92593

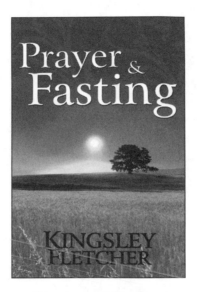

Prayer and Fasting

Dr. Kingsley Fletcher

Do you feel like your prayers are hitting the ceiling? Do you long to touch the heart of God like David, Esther, and Daniel? Are you ready for a breakthrough in your prayer life? Discover the synergistic power you can obtain by adding the element of fasting to your prayers. By incorporating Dr. Kingsley Fletcher's principles of prayer and fasting into your life, you can be infused with newfound purpose, be on fire for God, and experience incredible closeness with Him. Find out how prayer and fasting can bring revival and healing to your heart, your home, your church, your city, and even your nation.

ISBN: 978-0-88368-543-3 • Trade • 176 pages

WHITAKER HOUSE

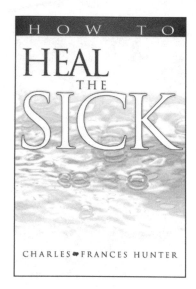

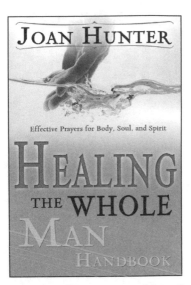

Healing the Whole Man Handbook:
Effective Prayers for Body, Soul, and Spirit
Joan Hunter

You can walk in divine health and healing. The secrets to God's words for healing and recovery are in this comprehensive, easy-to-follow guidebook containing powerful healing prayers that cover everything from abuse to yeast infections and everything in between.

Truly anointed with the gifts of healing, Joan Hunter has over thirty years of experience praying for the sick and brokenhearted and seeing them healed and set free. By following these step-by-step instructions and claiming God's promises, you can be healed, set free, and made totally whole—body, soul, and spirit!

ISBN: 978-0-88368-815-8 • Trade • 240 pages

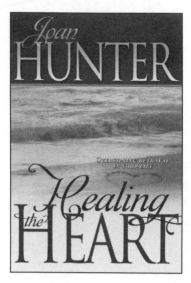

Healing the Heart:
Overcoming Betrayal in Your Life
Joan Hunter

For anyone who has ever been betrayed...
For anyone who has ever felt lost, abused, or abandoned...
For anyone who has ever suffered a broken heart...
THERE IS HEALING!
In this inspiring and life-changing book, Joan Hunter shares her challenging testimony of how she overcame rejection and the worst betrayal imaginable. No matter what your circumstances, God wants to minister to you through Joan's insights and practical advice.
On the cross, Jesus paid for more than your physical healing. He has also made provision for *Healing the Heart.*

ISBN: 978-0-88368-130-5 • Trade • 192 pages

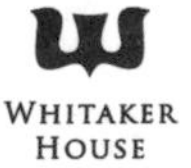

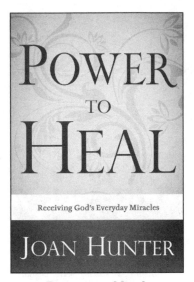

Power to Heal:
Experiencing the Miraculous
Joan Hunter

"Joan moves in the miraculous….The anointing of God rests upon her."
—Marilyn Hickey,
Founder and President, Marilyn Hickey Ministries

Joan Hunter reveals powerful truths about healing and being whole. Through this dynamic book, you will discover how to break generational curses, gain complete freedom from oppression, and end cycles of dependency. As you begin to understand what blocks healing, you will learn to walk in true forgiveness and break the devil's authority in your life. God has provided the miracle you need. Believe and receive today.

ISBN: 978-1-60374-111-8 • Trade • 224 pages

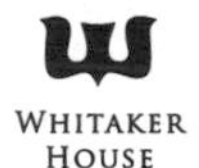

WHITAKER
HOUSE

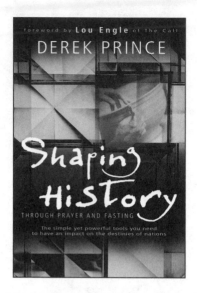

Shaping History through Prayer and Fasting
Derek Prince

The times we are living in are scary, to say the least, yet what we are facing isn't new. History is replete with violent episodes of unimaginable carnage and terror. And what did people do about them? The only thing they could do—they prayed! Best-selling author Derek Prince reveals how your prayers can make a real difference right now and into the future. Discover how to touch the heart of God through effective fasting and prayer—prayer that will change the world!

ISBN: 978-0-88368-773-4 • Trade • 192 pages

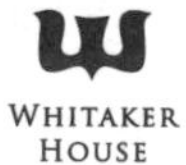